Herbal Tea

The Health Uses and History of Botanical Brews Across Civilizations and Time

Hourglass History

Table of Contents

Table of Contents

Introduction

In the very heart of humanity's past, entwined with its rituals, medicines, and daily sustenance, you find the ubiquitous presence of herbal teas. These are not just drinks, but potent symbols. They are emblems of the relationship between man and nature, representatives of the culture that partook in them, and sometimes, the very bonds that held communities together. At the intersection of botany, history, and health, herbal teas command a story, an odyssey, which transcends temporal boundaries and geographic divides.

But first, a definition: what are these 'herbal teas' we speak of so reverently? In truth, the term 'tea' when speaking of herbs is a bit of a misnomer. True tea—be it green, black, white, or oolong—comes from the Camellia sinensis plant. What we refer to as 'herbal tea' is more accurately an 'infusion' or 'tisane', a brew made from steeping herbs, flowers, roots, or other parts of a plant in hot water. Unlike the caffeine-infused cousins from the Camellia plant, herbal infusions don't always invigorate, but sometimes calm, heal, or simply delight the senses.

The roots of this ancient practice reach deep. Consider, for a moment, a time long past. Before agriculture's dawn, our ancestors were foragers. In the vast, untouched wilderness, they sought sustenance. But the land's flora was more than just a source of food. It was, crucially, a vast pharmacy. Every shrub or herb could be a remedy or poison. The line between the two was often thin, and discerning it was a matter of life or death. Thus began humanity's intimate dance with herbs.

The Mesopotamians were among the first to record their use of herbs, both culinary and medicinal. On clay tablets written in cuneiform, we find hints of their herbal wisdom, revealing the significance of plants like mint and licorice in their daily lives. Ancient Egyptian papyri, too, describe over 700 herbal remedies, including fennel and juniper, for various ailments.

China, with its ancient and enduring tradition of herbal medicine, elevated the use of herbal infusions to an art form. It was more than healing; it was a philosophical approach to balance and wellness. The Chinese pharmacopeia, 'Shennong Ben Cao Jing', penned over two millennia ago, extols the virtues of hundreds of herbs, detailing not only their healing properties but also their tastes, temperatures, and associated energies.

But as these botanical brews crisscrossed the globe, they took on cultural, economic, and even political significance. In Medieval Europe, herbs were integral to the monastic tradition. Monasteries were repositories of herbal knowledge, with monks tending elaborate gardens and crafting remedies for both their brethren and the lay community. The chamomile, soothing and fragrant, wasn't just a drink; in the hands of a Benedictine monk, it was an emblem of God's grace, a balm for both body and soul.

Yet, one might wonder, are these ancient remedies and infusions just relics of a bygone era, borne out of necessity and superseded by modern medicine? Far from it. Today, science increasingly echoes what our ancestors intuited through observation and experience. The antioxidants in rooibos, the anti-inflammatory properties of ginger, the calming effects of lavender – all stand up to rigorous scientific scrutiny.

However, let us not distill the essence of herbal teas merely into their chemical constituents. For, beyond the health benefits they bestow, they serve another, equally vital, function: a connection to our shared past. In the steam rising from a cup of elderflower infusion, we are invited to commune with an ancient Celt who might have believed in the tree's protective spirit. In the spicy embrace of cinnamon tea, we can traverse the old spice routes and feel the allure that once drove men to the ends of the earth.

The variety of these infusions is as vast as the tapestry of human culture itself. From the aromatic mint teas of the Maghreb to the bold maté of South America; from the delicate cherry blossom tisanes of Japan to the robust rooibos of South Africa - each brew is a chapter in the grand narrative of human civilization.

As we embark on this exploration, we are not just tracing the journey of herbal teas across time and space; we are mapping the contours of human history itself. The tales of empires, the interplay of cultures, the evolution of medicinal practices – they all converge in the humble cup of herbal brew.

Over the course of this book, we will explore the myriad health benefits and rich histories of thirty herbal teas. Each chapter will unveil a civilization's unique relationship with a particular herb, delving into their motivations for its use and its profound cultural and spiritual importance to them.

So, as you sip, ponder, and delve deeper into the following pages, remember: you're not just partaking in a drink. You're imbibing a tradition, a legacy, a story that has been millennia in the making. Welcome to the world of herbal teas, a world where history, health, and botany intertwine in the most delightful of dances.

Chamomile – Serenity in a Sip

Fragrance gentle, a sweet embrace,
Taste a journey to a tranquil place.
Beneath the moon, the plant does gleam,
Chamomile's magic, a dreamer's dream.

The Delicate Bloom: Matricaria Chamomilla
Petals of Light

Often mistaken for a daisy, the chamomile flower bears petals of purest white and a golden center, resembling our very sun. This dainty bloom, however, is more than just a pleasing aesthetic addition to gardens and meadows. Hidden in its delicate structure is a history of remedy, ritual, and refreshment.

The Rooted Wanderer

Chamomile, surprisingly, is not just one plant. Two types are predominantly used for making the tea we recognize today: the German chamomile (*Matricaria chamomilla*) and the Roman chamomile (*Chamaemelum nobile*). Though the two are distinct species, they share similar properties and have parallel histories of use across civilizations.

Origins and Etymology: More Than Just a Name
The Grecian Legacy

Chamomile's name is rooted in ancient Greece. Derived from the words "*chamos*" (ground) and "*melos*" (apple), it translates to 'ground apple'. This etymology paints a vivid imagery of the flower's habitat and hints at its aroma. But more than that, it ties the plant intrinsically to the cradle of Western civilization.

From Greek to Latin to Old French

Language, like chamomile, travels. From its Grecian roots, the name meandered into Latin as "chamomilla", which was subsequently adopted by Old French. The linguistic journey of chamomile is not just about shifts in nomenclature but is a reflection of the plant's movement across cultures, societies, and epochs.

Sensory Delight: Aroma and Taste

An Orchard in Bloom

Chamomile's aroma is reminiscent of a crisp apple. On a breezy autumn day, one can almost imagine walking through an orchard with fallen apples underfoot, releasing their fresh scent with each step. When steeped in hot water, the aroma transforms, becoming more floral, yet retaining that signature apple note.

The Liquid Lullaby

On the palate, chamomile is gentle. Its taste is subtly sweet with hints of earthiness. But it's not just the flavor that captures one's senses—it's the serenity it brings. Drinking chamomile tea is akin to being wrapped in a soft blanket, with lullabies whispered in the ears.

A Drink of Many Lands

The journey of chamomile is as meandering as the rivers of old. From Egypt to Rome, from medieval apothecaries to modern teacups, its gentle essence has been recognized and revered. As we delve into the depths of chamomile's tale, we are not just exploring a plant or a beverage, but a testament to humanity's age-old relationship with nature. Every sip, a whisper of the ages; every aroma, a scent-laden page from the annals of history.

Ancient Egypt: Civilization by the Nile

Sands of Time

Nestled between swathes of desert, the mighty Nile's fertile basin bore witness to one of humanity's most enigmatic and enduring civilizations: Ancient Egypt. Over millennia, Egypt's story is one of innovation, spirituality, and a profound relationship with the environment.

The Age of Pharaohs

Pharaohs, the god-kings, weren't just political leaders; they were the embodiment of Egypt's spiritual essence. Under their aegis, art, architecture, and agriculture thrived. Temples, pyramids, and obelisks weren't just stone structures but symbols of a civilization's deep yearning to understand and venerate the cosmos.

Chamomile in the Heart of the Desert

Brewed in Gold

To the Ancient Egyptians, chamomile was not merely a plant but a gift from the gods. Documentations, such as the

Ebers Papyrus - one of the oldest and most comprehensive medical treatises from Ancient Egypt - list chamomile for its therapeutic properties.

Spiritual Significance

In a land where the spiritual and physical realms intermingled freely, chamomile assumed a position of reverence. This was not just a flower but a symbol. It was believed to be an offering to the Sun God, Ra, for his blessings. In the intricate Egyptian hieroglyphs, chamomile appeared as a motif, signifying the cycle of life, death, and rebirth.

The Pharaoh's Cup: The Ritual Brew

More than Just a Drink

For Ancient Egyptians, drinking chamomile was not a casual affair. It was a ritual. The golden hue of the brew symbolized the mighty sun setting over the Nile. Ingesting it was believed to imbibe the drinker with the Sun's vitality. The Pharaohs, in their divine wisdom, often consumed chamomile before significant events, seeking blessings and clarity.

Healing Elixirs

Beyond the spiritual, chamomile had tangible, therapeutic applications. Ancient Egyptian physicians prescribed chamomile for various ailments, from digestive disorders to fever and pain. The flower's potent anti-inflammatory properties made it an essential part of their medical repertoire.

From the Past to the Present: Chamomile's Enduring Legacy

Modern Revelations

Centuries have passed, yet chamomile's appeal remains undiminished. Today, scientific studies affirm what the Ancient Egyptians inherently understood. Chamomile is rich in antioxidants, particularly quercetin, which plays a pivotal role in fighting inflammation and maintaining cellular health.

Sleep's Gentle Embrace

One of the most lauded benefits of chamomile in our frenzied modern era is its ability to induce sleep. The compound apigenin in chamomile binds to specific brain receptors, promoting sleepiness and reducing insomnia.

Digestive Harmony

Just as the Ancient Egyptian texts indicated, chamomile's benefits for the digestive system are significant. It alleviates symptoms of indigestion, gas, and even irritable bowel syndrome, bringing a sense of calm to turbulent stomachs.

Precautions and Interactions

Not Everyone's Cup of Tea

Though chamomile is generally safe, some individuals might exhibit allergic reactions, particularly those allergic to plants in the Asteraceae family. Symptoms can range from skin rashes to, in rare cases, anaphylaxis.

When blending chamomile with other herbal teas, it's crucial to be aware of potential interactions. For instance, combined with sedative herbs like valerian or hops, the sleep-inducing effects can amplify, potentially leading to excessive drowsiness.

Conclusion: A Sip Through Time

As we journey from the past to the present, chamomile's story is more than just about a tea. It's about civilizations, beliefs, and the age-old human desire for healing and connection. On the banks of the Nile, under the shadow of the pyramids, chamomile found its sacred space. Today, as we hold our cups, steaming with the golden brew, we aren't just drinking a tea; we're partaking in a ritual that spans millennia. We're sipping history, one soothing gulp at a time.

Peppermint - The Cool Breeze

A burst of chill, a zesty spree,
Peppermint's dance, wild and free.
Winter's touch on a summer's day,
Reviving the soul in every way.

The world of herbal teas boasts a plethora of infusions, each with its own story and identity. And yet, few possess the vivacity and unmistakable allure of peppermint. It is a tea that captures the very essence of invigoration—a gust of crisp air, a brush of cool wind on a summer's day. From where does this sensation spring? From a seemingly unassuming herb that, upon closer observation, unfurls layers of history, botany, and cultural significance.

To embark on the journey of peppermint tea is to trace the steps of *Mentha x piperita*—the botanical embodiment of peppermint. A natural hybrid of watermint and spearmint, peppermint is no ordinary mint. Its vibrancy, its assertiveness, its zing—it all points to a plant that is both a product of nature's whimsy and human cultivation.

Origins: A Twist of Fate and Botany

Though peppermint's parent plants, watermint and spearmint, have been known since ancient times, peppermint, as we recognize it, is relatively newer. It wasn't the meticulous work of an ancient botanist nor the deliberate cross-breeding by an early cultivator that brought this plant into existence. Instead, nature herself played matchmaker. By some quirk of botanical fate, the watermint and spearmint plants grew close enough to cross-pollinate, and the result was a herbaceous prodigy: peppermint. This serendipitous birth would go on to change culinary and medicinal landscapes across continents.

While the precise geographic origin of peppermint remains debated, the general consensus aligns with its emergence in Europe, later migrating across diverse terrains and climes.

The Name: Whence Peppermint?

Peppermint's etymology carries with it echoes of its characteristics. Derived from the Latin "piper," reminiscent of the spiciness of black pepper, and "mentha," attributed to Minthe, a water nymph in Greek mythology transformed into a plant by Persephone out of jealousy, the name encapsulates both the plant's zing and its aqueous origins.

Minthe's tragic transformation has been immortalized in several Grecian tales, where her fate was sealed by her own beauty and allure. Just as Minthe was irresistible to Hades, peppermint, too, possesses an alluring charm, drawing in those who chance upon its aroma.

The Aroma: An Olfactory Symphony

Imagine for a moment, standing amidst a field of peppermint, the air alive with its scent. It's an olfactory symphony—an initial burst of coolness, followed by subtle earthy undertones, rounded off with a hint of sweetness. The aroma is so potent that even a gentle brush against its leaves releases a wave of refreshing fragrance. This aromatic richness isn't merely a treat for the senses but a testament to the plant's rich reserve of essential oils, with menthol being the most dominant.

The Palate's Play: Tasting the Breeze

To describe the taste of peppermint tea is akin to capturing the sensation of a breeze on one's face. The initial sip introduces a cooling sensation, a crispness that awakens the palate. Then, as the liquid swirls, there's a hint of sweetness, a gentle counterbalance to its cool nature. The aftertaste lingers, a gentle reminder of the meadows and gardens where peppermint thrives.

But beyond the sensation lies chemistry. The cooling effect can be attributed to menthol, which interacts with the body's cold-sensitive receptors, creating a sensation of coolness without an actual drop in temperature.

The Persian Pas de Deux with Peppermint

The air in ancient Persia was replete with a mix of fragrances—cedarwood from the massive palaces, saffron from the sprawling fields, and, of course, peppermint. The verdant expanse of Persia provided an ideal milieu for the mint to flourish, but it was the Persians themselves who elevated the herb to an elixir of luxury and wellness.

The Tapestry of Persia

Before we delve into peppermint's role in Persia, let's unfold the grand tapestry of the civilization itself. Persia, today's Iran, was home to one of the world's most advanced and luxurious ancient cultures. This was a land where great emperors, like Cyrus and Darius, ruled vast territories, where the architectural marvels such as Persepolis stood tall, and where Zoroastrianism influenced thoughts and philosophies.

Sprawling between the Caspian Sea and the Persian Gulf, this terrain of contrasts—deserts, fertile plains, and high mountains—was united under the banner of the Achaemenid Empire. As the empire expanded, so did its network of roads, facilitating the flow of goods, including herbs and spices, setting the stage for peppermint's prominence.

The Persian Peppermint Pantheon

In ancient Persia, gardens were not mere spaces of leisure. They were a testament to man's ability to harness nature, to create order amidst the wilderness. The *pairidaēza* (paradise) garden, a walled enclosure, was a Persian concept and it was within these verdant expanses that peppermint thrived.

Mint, in its various forms, was no stranger to the Persians. But peppermint, with its vivacious vigor and aromatic aura, found a special place in the Persian culinary and medicinal lexicon. Consumed in teas or used as a fragrant herb in their opulent feasts, peppermint was a signifier of luxury, much like saffron or rosewater.

Sacred Herb of Ahura Mazda?

While there isn't direct evidence linking peppermint to Zoroastrian rituals, herbs and plants held a significant place in the religion. It's plausible that peppermint, given its prominence in daily life, might have been associated with some rituals or medicinal practices tied to the faith. As the worshippers of Ahura Mazda sought asha (truth and order), they looked to nature for signs and solutions. Herbs were considered divine gifts, each with its purpose and potency. Peppermint, with its refreshing properties, could easily be imagined as a herb bestowing clarity and vigor.

Health in a Cup: The Ancient Wellness Elixir

The Persians were no strangers to the world of medicinal herbs. The likes of Avicenna, a Persian polymath, penned down extensive tracts on the use of herbs and their health benefits. While peppermint may not have found specific mention in his works, the broader Persian medical tradition recognized mint's therapeutic properties. Peppermint tea was not merely a beverage of refreshment but a draught of wellness. Its cooling nature was believed to balance the body's humors, particularly bile. Consumed post feasts, it acted as a digestive. On torrid days, it promised respite from the heat.

Modern Health Attributes

Transitioning from ancient scrolls and oral traditions to modern clinical trials, peppermint has held its ground as a herb of myriad benefits. Digestion, for one, has remained its forte. Modern studies suggest that peppermint oil can ease symptoms of irritable bowel syndrome. Its antispasmodic properties help relax the gut muscles.

Moreover, menthol, the primary constituent of peppermint, is known to act as a decongestant. A cup of peppermint tea during colds or respiratory infections can clear nasal passages and soothe sore throats. Its anti-inflammatory properties, too, come to the fore, making it a balm for headaches and migraines.

Interactions and Cautions

Like all things potent, peppermint comes with its caveats. Consumed in excess, it might exacerbate heartburn or lead to nausea. Those with a predisposition to acid reflux or GERD might want to exercise caution.

When it comes to blending, peppermint is both a collaborator and a dominant force. It pairs harmoniously with herbs like chamomile, offering a blend of calm and clarity. However, its potency might overshadow more delicate herbs or render certain combinations too cooling.

In the Blend of Times

Peppermint, in its journey from the ancient Persian gardens to modern cups, has witnessed winds of change. And through it all, it has remained, not as a mere herb, but as a symbol—a reminder of nature's bounty and of Persian opulence.

Hibiscus - The Ruby of the Herbal Realm

Delicately plucked from the shrubs of tropical regions, the hibiscus flower, with its radiant crimson hue, stands as an emblem of vibrancy and vivacity. Not merely a sight for sore eyes, these petals, when steeped, produce a tea rich in color and character, quite unlike any other. It is not just a beverage; it is an odyssey that connects continents, cultures, and epochs.

A Botanical Marvel

The hibiscus plant, botanically christened *Hibiscus sabdariffa*, is a wonder in itself. It's not merely one species but a vast genus, housing over two hundred species. Ranging from annuals to perennials, from woody shrubs to small trees, the variations are myriad. Yet, when it comes to our coveted brew, it is the *Hibiscus sabdariffa*, specifically its calyces, that reigns supreme.

But, how did this tropical wonder spread its roots (both literally and metaphorically) far and wide? There's a history, threaded with migrations, discoveries, and of course, human insatiable thirst for the new and the novel.

Origins - A Tale of Continents

The tapestry of the hibiscus's journey is intricate, to say the least. Native to West Africa, its vibrant petals might have danced to the balmy African winds, but its reputation soon reached far shores.

The etymology itself is a tapestry woven of Greek threads. Deriving from the Greek word 'hibiskos', which was used to refer to marshmallow, the name is somewhat of a misnomer. For the hibiscus is no marsh plant. But, such is the nature of names—they stick, sometimes for reasons lost in the annals of time.

An Olfactory and Gustatory Expedition

Before we proceed, let's engage in an exercise—a sensory sojourn, if you will. Close your eyes and imagine a steaming cup of hibiscus tea. Its deep ruby hue is the first signifier of its uniqueness. But wait, let's not get ahead of ourselves. Before the taste, comes the aroma.

The fragrance is distinct—floral, naturally, but there's an underlying tang. It's not pungent but rather invigorating. This is not a scent that lulls; it's one that enlivens.

Now, take a sip. The first note that hits is tartness, akin to cranberries. But, much like a symphony that unfolds in movements, the flavor profile evolves. There's sweetness, a subtle underbelly to the tart top notes. It's this dance between sweet and sour that makes hibiscus tea an experience, not just a beverage. And as it trickles down, there's a warmth, a vibrancy, a certain tropical lushness that lingers.

Palette of the Tropics

With the sensual experience elucidated, let's delve back into its storied past. This is not a tale of a solitary land but rather a mosaic of cultures and terrains. Hibiscus, despite its African origins, soon found itself in Asian soils. India, in particular, embraced it, not just as a beverage but as an integral component of its traditional medicine system, Ayurveda.

Asia aside, the flower made its way to the European landscape. How? Through the intricate web of trade routes. Merchants, enticed by its vivid hue and unique taste, saw potential—both medicinal and culinary. And, as they say, the rest is history.

Hibiscus in the Heart of Sudan

From the intersection of the Blue and White Nile, the Sudanese civilization rose, with a history both poignant and profound. It was here, amidst the swirling dust and the vastness of the Sahara, that the hibiscus found more than just fertile ground—it found a home, a culture, and a people who cherished it.

Sudan: Where Civilizations Converged

The story of Sudan is one of confluence. At the junction of Africa and the Middle East, Sudan had been a cradle for diverse civilizations: from the ancient Nubians to the Islamic caliphates, from the fur-trading sultanates to the British colonial empire. To capture its essence, one must envision the grand temples of Meroë, the Islamic frescoes of old mosques, and the bustling markets of Khartoum.

Beyond its strategic location, the Nile provided life to Sudan. Its annual inundation deposited rich silt on the banks, making it a fertile ground for agriculture, and, among its bounties, was the Hibiscus.

The Sudanese and their 'Karkade'

In Sudan, hibiscus tea isn't just another beverage; it's *karkade*, a drink deeply embedded in the Sudanese psyche. But to reduce *karkade* merely to its status as a popular beverage would be to oversimplify its significance.

Imagine, if you will, the sprawling bazaars of Omdurman in the late afternoon. The call to prayer echoes in the distance, and as the day's heat begins its slow descent into a cooler evening, large copper pots simmer with deep red *karkade*. Its aroma, both tangy and floral, wafts through the air, inviting passersby to take a momentary respite from their routines.

However, it wasn't just the thirst-quenching attributes of *karkade* that endeared it to the Sudanese. It played—and continues to play—a ceremonial role. At weddings, births, and religious festivities, *karkade* was more than a mere drink; it was a symbol of hospitality, of shared moments, and of the Sudanese penchant for communal celebrations.

Spiritual Elixirs?

Was there a spiritual element to *karkade*? In Sudan, the lines between the religious, the cultural, and the daily often blur. While not directly associated with religious rites, *karkade*, due to its prominence in festivities, often found itself in the backdrop of religious celebrations, especially during Ramadan. As the sun set and the day's fast came to an end, families often broke their fast with a refreshing glass of chilled *karkade*.

Modern Rediscoveries and Health Implications

The world has woken up to what the Sudanese knew for centuries: that this ruby-red concoction isn't just pleasing to the palate but has a plethora of health benefits.

Modern science affirms that hibiscus tea can aid in lowering blood pressure, thereby benefiting heart health. Its rich antioxidant properties mean it combats free radicals in the body, reducing the risk of chronic diseases. Furthermore, there have been studies suggesting its role in supporting liver health and promoting weight loss. In the fight against bacterial infections, too, *karkade* stands its ground, showcasing antibacterial properties.

However, like any substance, moderation is key. Consumed in excess, hibiscus tea can have a diuretic effect. For those on medication, especially those for hypertension, there can be potential interactions. Additionally, due to its potential to lower blood sugar levels, those on diabetes medication should also exercise caution.

Blend and Harmony

One of the beautiful aspects of hibiscus tea is its adaptability. In blends, it complements and contrasts in delightful ways. With its tartness, it can balance sweeter herbs like licorice or stevia. When paired with spices like cinnamon or cloves, it adds a fruitiness that enlivens the blend.

However, blending isn't just about flavors; it's about the synergy of effects. When combined with herbs known for their calming effects, like chamomile or lavender, hibiscus can offer a relaxation blend. But, when blended with invigorating herbs like ginger or mint, it transforms into an energizing concoction.

In essence, the tale of hibiscus in Sudan is not merely one of a beverage. It's a tale of a people, of a culture, and of the myriad ways in which nature intertwines with our lives. As we sip on our *karkade*, whether in the heart of Khartoum or in a distant corner of the globe, we partake in a tradition, an experience, and a history that reminds us of the timelessness of human connections.

Ginger - The Fiery Root of Asia's History

Aroma entices, taste does inspire,
Rooted deep, it's nature's fire.
Ginger's essence, in tea does blend,
A timeless story, with no end.

The Plant and its Bold Persona

In the dense, moist tropical forests of Southeast Asia, amidst tall trees and a symphony of birds, a herb grows close to the ground, unassuming and easily overlooked. This is Zingiber officinale, better known as ginger, a rhizome with a presence as sharp and piercing as its flavor.

In botanical terms, ginger isn't a root but a rhizome, a horizontal stem from which shoots and roots grow, often sneaking underground. Above ground, its reed-like stems stretch up, crowned with narrow, green leaves. By late summer, the plant blooms with delicate, yellow-green flowers, tinged with purple edges. Yet, the real magic lies beneath the soil.

From Southeast Asia to the World: Ginger's Odyssey

Though today it thrives in many tropical locales, ginger's origins can be traced back to maritime Southeast Asia. Ancient texts, botany, and linguistics collectively point towards the region encompassing the islands of Java, Sumatra, Borneo, and the Malay Peninsula as the native home of ginger.

One of humanity's most ancient cultivated plants, ginger embarked on an odyssey, traveling through trade routes and entering ancient scripts. By the time of the Roman Empire, ginger was being imported in significant quantities into the Mediterranean from India.

Etymology: A Linguistic Journey

The word 'ginger' echoes through time, indicative of the plant's extensive journey across cultures and geographies. Derived from the Middle English 'gingivere', it finds its roots in the Old French 'gingibre', which was adapted from the Latin 'zingiberis'. This Latin term, however, owes its origin to the Greek 'zingiberis', which was borrowed from Prakrit (Middle Indic) 'singabera', meaning 'shaped like a horn'.

The lineage of the name itself, winding back through European, Greek, and Indic cultures, is a testimony to ginger's vast cultural journey.

The Olfactory and Gustatory Experience

Ginger presents an olfactory enigma. At first, the nose detects a woody freshness, reminiscent of lemony pine. But as one delves deeper, there's the hint of warmth, a spicy resonance that feels comforting, invigorating.

On the palate, ginger is a paradox. It begins with a mildly sweet touch, evoking thoughts of delicate floral nectars. But, within moments, the sweetness is overshadowed by a warm, peppery spiciness. This heat, both surprising and invigorating, is due to the presence of gingerol, a natural chemical that also imparts several of ginger's renowned health properties.

From its tropical heartland in Southeast Asia, ginger ventured forth into human civilization, becoming a mainstay in culinary and medicinal traditions, influencing and being influenced by the cultural fabric of societies. Now, as we trace its journey into the annals of Chinese history, we'll delve deeper into its significance, uses, and the myriad ways it has intertwined with human narratives.

The Middle Kingdom and Its Timeless Allure

One cannot embark upon a discussion about ginger in the realm of history without first setting foot into the world of ancient China – a civilization where rivers nurtured lands, and legends wove themselves into the tapestry of reality. The Yellow River, often termed the "Cradle of Chinese Civilization," bore witness to the rise of dynasties that not only shaped the fate of millions but also sowed the seeds of cultural and culinary traditions that are revered even today.

Ginger in the Chronicles of Ancient China

Within the vast expanse of Chinese history, ginger has been more than a mere root. It's been a medicinal wonder, a culinary mainstay, and at times, a symbol of vitality and warmth. The earliest mentions can be traced back to the classics of Chinese medicine. The legendary "Shennong Ben Cao Jing," a pharmacopeia penned under the mythical Emperor Shennong's guidance, extols ginger's virtues, placing it among the upper echelon of herbs that bestow longevity and vigor.

A Brew of Wellness: Ginger Tea in Dynastic Eras

While ginger graced many a recipe in ancient Chinese culinary traditions, its avatar as a tea held a special place. Boiled ginger water, sometimes sweetened with a touch of honey or jaggery, was a common remedy for colds and respiratory ailments. During the chilly winters, especially in the northern realms of the empire, ginger tea was seen as a shield against the biting cold, its warmth believed to rejuvenate the Qi – the life force.

It's worth noting that while tea, as a beverage, rose to prominence during the Tang dynasty, herbal infusions had been in practice long before. Ginger, with its intrinsic heat, was often the primary ingredient in these infusions, believed to expel cold and dampness from the body.

The Spiritual Essence of Ginger

In the spiritual and philosophical realm, Taoism, an indigenous Chinese religion, often emphasized harmony with the Tao, a principle that is the source, pattern, and substance of everything that exists. The concept of Yin and Yang, representing the interdependence of opposites, was central to this belief system.

Ginger, with its warming properties, was seen as a yang food. Consuming it, especially during Yin-dominated periods (like the cold winters), was believed to restore balance. In this regard, ginger tea was more than just a beverage; it was an elixir that harmonized the spirit, body, and the universe.

Modern Marvels: Ginger's Contemporary Healing Touch

Fast forward to the present day, and ginger remains a beloved ingredient in Chinese households and Traditional Chinese Medicine (TCM) practices. But its acclaim is no longer limited to China; the modern world has embraced ginger tea for its myriad health benefits.

1. **Digestive Aid**: One of the most well-acknowledged benefits of ginger is its ability to alleviate gastrointestinal irritation, stimulate saliva, and suppress gastric contractions as food and fluids move through the GI tract.

2. **Anti-inflammatory and Antioxidative Properties**: Gingerol, the bioactive substance in ginger, has powerful anti-inflammatory and antioxidant effects.

3. **Combatting Nausea**: From morning sickness to chemotherapy-induced nausea, ginger has shown promise as a potential remedy.

4. **Fighting off Colds and Flu**: Much like the ancient Chinese believed, modern studies suggest that ginger might indeed help in reducing the symptoms of colds and flu.

A Note of Caution: The Potential Side-Effects

While ginger tea is generally considered safe for consumption, excessive intake can lead to adverse effects, including heartburn, diarrhea, and abdominal discomfort. Additionally, ginger's blood-thinning properties mean that it should be consumed judiciously by those on blood-thinning medications.

The Dance of Herbs: Ginger's Interactions in Blends

In the world of herbal teas, blending is an art, a science, and sometimes, a serendipitous discovery. Ginger, with its robust flavor profile, can either dominate or complement when paired with other herbs.

1. **With Turmeric**: This blend amplifies anti-inflammatory benefits, with both herbs having a rich history in traditional medicine.

2. **With Lemongrass**: This combination, popular in many Southeast Asian cuisines, offers a refreshing zing, ideal for warm climates.

3. **With Licorice Root**: While ginger heats, licorice cools, providing a balanced blend, often used in TCM to harmonize other herbs in the mix.

The story of ginger is as much about its journey through time as it is about its transformative impact on health and wellness. From the dynastic eras of ancient China to the bustling metropolises of the 21st century, ginger has remained an enduring, warming presence – a testament to nature's timeless gifts to humanity.

Echinacea – The Verdant Healer of the Prairies

Purple petals, a cone-like heart,
Echinacea stands beautifully apart.
Nature's sentinel, tall and grand,
A healer from the prairie land.

From the Heart of North America: Echinacea's Roots

Lying beneath the vast skies of North America's midwestern plains and meadows is a botanical marvel, Echinacea. These daisy-like flowers, with their proud conical centers, are not just an aesthetic delight but have been a repository of healing for ages. Their origins are deep-seated in the soils of the prairies, from the wild expanse of eastern and central North America, where they grow wild and free.

Echinacea: Etymology and Its Significance

The name Echinacea finds its roots in the Greek word "echinos," which means "hedgehog" or "sea urchin." This peculiar naming stems from the spiky appearance of the plant's central cone, reminiscent of the sharp spines of a hedgehog or the undulating arms of a sea urchin. The etymology itself provides an intriguing glimpse into the human propensity for linking the known with the unknown, drawing parallels between the familiar creatures of their surroundings and the newfound botanical wonders.

The Fragrance and Flavor: A Sensory Journey

If you were to take a stroll through a meadow at the height of summer, the mild, sweet aroma of Echinacea might just beckon you. Its scent is not overpowering; rather, it whispers gently of earth and sunshine, a subtle reminder of nature's embrace.

Brew a cup of Echinacea tea, and its flavor profile would be equally gentle on the palate: subtly sweet, with earthy undertones. Some have even described it as having a tongue-tingling sensation, a slight numbing that is distinctive but not overwhelming.

Echinacea's Ancestral Legacy

Nature's best-kept secrets often lie in plain sight. Echinacea is one such treasure. Before it caught the attention of the broader world, it had been a cornerstone in the traditions of those who first roamed North America's sprawling landscapes.

Native American tribes, particularly those of the plains, held Echinacea in high regard, not just for its curative properties but as a symbol of the untamed spirit of the land. To understand the depth of Echinacea's significance, it's essential to delve into the cultures and beliefs of the Plains Tribes.

One might wonder, why Echinacea? Amongst the myriad of flora across the prairies, what made this particular plant stand out? The answer, as with many historical conundrums, is a blend of practicality and spirituality. The tribes of the plains, in their deep connection with the land, learned to read nature's signs, turning to Echinacea as a trusted ally against ailments. Yet, its importance was not merely medicinal; it was a bridge between the earthly realm and the spiritual world.

The Plains Tribes: A Snapshot of an Era

The Great Plains, stretching from the Mississippi River to the Rocky Mountains, was more than just vast expanses of grassland. It was a vibrant tapestry of cultures, languages, and traditions – a testament to the indomitable spirit of the Plains Tribes. Comprising nations such as the Lakota, Cheyenne, Arapaho, and Comanche, these nomadic tribes epitomized adaptation and resilience in the face of nature's harsh whims.

Their lifeways, dictated by the rhythms of seasons and migrations, revolved around the buffalo. These majestic beasts provided sustenance, tools, and shelter, but their importance went beyond the material. They were revered spiritual symbols, a bridge between the terrestrial and the ethereal. Yet, alongside the buffalo, the Plains Tribes had another, less conspicuous ally: the Echinacea plant.

Echinacea's Role in Traditional Medicine

For these tribes, the vast prairies were more than hunting grounds; they were nature's pharmacy. Among the myriad of herbs and plants, Echinacea stood out, not just for its vivid appearance but for its healing properties.

A Panacea for the Prairie-Dweller

Echinacea, known by various indigenous names, was recognized for its ability to treat a plethora of ailments.

From soothing toothaches and snake bites to dressing wounds and countering infections, its applications were manifold. The root, rich in medicinal compounds, was particularly prized. Tribes would chew it directly or brew it into a potent tea, trusting in its curative prowess.

Beyond the Physical: Spiritual Significance

Echinacea was not just a physical remedy; it held spiritual significance for many Plains Tribes. Much like other elements of their environment, the tribes saw a deeper, spiritual dimension to this plant.

Echinacea in Rituals and Ceremonies

For certain tribes, Echinacea played a role in sacred ceremonies. It was believed that the plant could help bridge the gap between the physical realm and the spirit world. Consuming Echinacea tea or using the plant in rituals was a way to seek clarity, guidance, or protection from ancestral spirits.

Echinacea in the Modern Age: A Resurgence of Ancient Wisdom

With the westward expansion and the subsequent collision of cultures, many indigenous practices were sidelined or forgotten. However, as the 20th century dawned, a newfound interest in herbal remedies saw Echinacea being rediscovered by the broader world.

Modern Uses and Health Benefits

Today, Echinacea is heralded for its immune-boosting properties. As a herbal supplement, it has found its way into the modern pharmacopeia, recommended for cold and flu prevention. Studies have also hinted at its anti-inflammatory properties, making it a natural remedy for skin conditions and minor wounds.

While the Plains Tribes might have intuitively understood the benefits of Echinacea, contemporary science is now validating and expanding upon that ancient knowledge.

Potential Side Effects

While Echinacea's health benefits are numerous, it's essential to understand its limitations and potential side effects. Modern research suggests that prolonged consumption can lead to nausea, dizziness, or even allergic reactions in some individuals. It's always advised to consult with a health professional before incorporating Echinacea or any herbal remedy into one's regimen.

The Art of Blending: Echinacea's Interactions with Other Herbal Teas

Herbal tea blending is both an art and science. When Echinacea joins the mix, its potent properties can enhance or modify the effects of other herbs.

For instance, when paired with elderberry, another immune-boosting herb, their combined effect is believed to be synergistic in bolstering the body's defenses. However, when mixed with herbs like St John's Wort, which can stimulate the immune system, there might be an over-amplification of effects.

Understanding these interactions is crucial. Blending Echinacea with complementary herbs can harness its benefits, but care should be taken to avoid unintended side effects.

Echinacea's Timeless Legacy

Echinacea's story is one of enduring significance. From the hands of Plains Tribes' shamans to the shelves of modern apothecaries, its journey speaks volumes about humanity's continual quest for healing and harmony. As we sip on a warm cup of Echinacea tea, we're not just consuming a herbal concoction; we're partaking in a tradition that spans centuries, cultures, and continents. In Echinacea, the legacy of the Plains Tribes lives on, reminding us of nature's boundless generosity and the timeless bond between humans and the land they inhabit.

Rooibos - The Red Elixir of the Cape

From arid lands, a taste so fine,
Rooibos shines, in every line.
A melody of warmth, rich and deep,
Memories of Africa, in every steep.

The Unique Botany of Rooibos: A Plant Unlike Any Other

Found primarily in the Cederberg region of South Africa, *Aspalathus linearis* is no ordinary shrub. Rooibos (pronounced "ROY-boss") means "red bush" in Afrikaans, and it's not hard to understand why. When its needle-like leaves are crushed and oxidized, they take on a deep red hue, reminiscent of the very soil from which they spring.

Yet, this plant, with its wiry stems and vibrant color, thrives in conditions where many others would surrender. The sandy slopes and craggy mountains of the Cederberg provide a unique combination of climate and geography, essential for the Rooibos plant's growth. This specificity, this demand for a particular slice of the earth, makes commercial cultivation of Rooibos a meticulous endeavor.

From Afrikaans Roots: The Etymology of Rooibos

The name "Rooibos" is as much a descriptor as it is a tribute to the Afrikaans-speaking people who popularized its use. In Afrikaans, "rooi" translates to red, and "bos" to bush, thus giving us the term "red bush". But the journey of naming this beverage is more than just translation—it is a tapestry woven from the threads of colonization, linguistic evolution, and indigenous knowledge.

Rooibos' Symphony: Aromas and Tastes

Rooibos is a tea that demands attention, not by force, but through the sheer depth of its character. A sip is an invitation to the rugged landscapes of the Cederberg, with all their wild, untamed beauty.

The Aromatic Ballet

Hold a cup of brewed Rooibos to your nose, and you're immediately met with a melody of scents. There's the earthy undertone, reminiscent of the dry soil from which the plant emerges. Yet, layered on top are sweeter notes—vanilla, perhaps a touch of caramel or honey. It's a heady mix, one that promises complexity.

On the Tongue

Rooibos does not betray its aromatic promises. As the liquid touches the palate, it dances—light, yet profound. Initially, there's the sweetness, but it's not cloying. It's balanced by a slight nuttiness, a touch of malty richness. Then, as it settles, the earthy tones emerge, grounding the entire experience. It's a tea that lingers, not just on the tongue, but in the memory.

The Enigma of Rooibos

To consider Rooibos merely as a tea would be to do it a disservice. It is a liquid tapestry of history, geography, and culture. Each cup holds the essence of a region, a reflection of the rugged Cederberg mountains, and the ancient sands that cradle the roots of the *Aspalathus linearis*.

Echoes from the Past: The Khoisan Civilization

To traverse the sands of time, journeying back thousands of years, is to encounter the indigenous Khoisan peoples—the original inhabitants of Southern Africa. These were not a singular people but a tapestry of culturally distinct groups, mainly the pastoral Khoikhoi and the hunter-gatherer San.

Language and Legacy

Khoisan languages, characterized by their distinct click consonants, are among the most ancient on our planet, giving voice to tales that predate recorded history. Their rock art, found extensively across the region, stands as a testament to their artistic prowess, their spiritual insights, and their intimate knowledge of the land and its bounties.

The Brew of the Bush: Khoisan and Rooibos

Long before the European settlers arrived on the shores of Southern Africa, the Khoisan had discovered the magical properties of the *Aspalathus linearis* plant. Rooibos was not just a drink—it was a tradition, an integral component of their way of life.

Harvest and Preparation

The Khoisan's method of preparing Rooibos was meticulous, rooted in generations of practice. Using primitive tools, they would ascend the mountainous terrains, seeking out the young Rooibos shoots. Once harvested, these were bound together and beaten using wooden hammers, facilitating the oxidation that gave the tea its distinctive red hue. Post this, they were sun-dried, infusing the leaves with the warmth of the African sun.

More than a Beverage

To the Khoisan, Rooibos was not just about quenching thirst. It was communal, an experience shared around fires, under the vastness of the starlit sky. There was an almost reverential aspect to its consumption—a celebration of nature's bounties and the ancestral knowledge that had led them to this herbal treasure.

The Spiritual Essence of Rooibos

Many San legends and myths surround the Rooibos plant, tying it to the very creation of their world. While detailed records of these tales are scant—owing to the oral nature of their tradition—it's evident that Rooibos occupied a sacred space in their cosmology.

Healing and Harmony

Beyond the spiritual, the Khoisan revered Rooibos for its healing properties. They intuited what science would later confirm: Rooibos was a balm, a remedy. From alleviating stomach cramps to providing relief from allergies, the tea was their go-to medicinal solution, a testament to their profound understanding of botany and natural healing.

Rooibos in Modern Times: From the Cape to the Globe

The journey of Rooibos, from the rugged terrains of the Cederberg to the teacups of global connoisseurs, is nothing short of remarkable. Today, it's celebrated not just for its unique taste but also for its myriad health benefits.

Health Benefits: A Brew of Wellbeing

Modern science, with its instruments of precision, has only reaffirmed what the Khoisan have known for centuries. Rooibos is a powerhouse of antioxidants, which combat free radicals, potentially reducing the risk of diseases. Moreover, being caffeine-free, it's a preferred choice for many seeking a calming beverage. Additionally, studies suggest that Rooibos can potentially aid cardiovascular health, improve skin condition, and even support weight loss.

Potential Side Effects

While Rooibos is generally considered safe for most people, it's not without its cautions. Some individuals might experience liver issues if consumed in excessive amounts. It also contains certain compounds that might act as estrogen, hence those with hormone-sensitive conditions should consume it judiciously.

When Rooibos Mingles: Interactions in a Blend

In the vast world of herbal teas, blending has become an art form. Rooibos, with its distinct profile, offers a palette that can enhance or be enhanced when combined with other herbs.

The Symphony of Blends

The nutty, earthy tones of Rooibos can complement the sharpness of mint or the sweetness of chamomile, creating a multi-layered beverage experience. When blended with hibiscus, another antioxidant-rich herb, the result is a tangy, refreshing drink that amplifies the health benefits.

However, blending isn't just about flavors; it's also about interactions. For instance, while Rooibos itself is caffeine-free, blending it with green or black tea would introduce caffeine into the mix.

In Conclusion: Rooibos, The Khoisan, and the Continuum of Time

As we sip on a cup of Rooibos today, we partake in a tradition that is millennia old, one that bridges the gap between the ancient and the contemporary. The Khoisan, with their profound wisdom, have bequeathed to us a legacy—a tea that is as much about health as it is about history.

Yet, it's more than just a beverage. It's a testament to humanity's enduring bond with nature, a bond that the Khoisan nurtured and celebrated. In Rooibos, we find the echoes of their laughter, their songs, and their tales—a red thread that weaves through time, connecting us all.

Lemongrass - Energizing Zest of the East

Tall and slender, green blades stand,
Lemongrass grows on sun-kissed land.
Amidst nature's orchestra, it plays its part,
A fragrant rhythm, a work of art.

The Green Scepter: Anatomy of Lemongrass

Dwelling primarily in the tropics, the *Cymbopogon* plant, popularly christened as lemongrass, is not just another green in the vast tapestry of flora. Its tall, slender, fibrous stalks carry an aroma so distinct, a fragrance so revitalizing, that its recognition is immediate. Its green and white blades, like Nature's own paintbrushes, paint a picture of the regions they grace.

Origins: From Obscurity to Luminescence

To trace the journey of lemongrass is to embark on a voyage through time and cultures. While its exact origin remains shrouded in the mists of antiquity, historical botanical consensus places its cradle in Southern India and Sri Lanka. However, it wasn't content staying rooted. Lemongrass embarked on its own journey, making its way across the vast Asian continent, adapting, thriving, and weaving itself into the fabric of diverse cultures.

Etymology: Naming the Fragrant Reed

The moniker 'lemongrass' is relatively self-explanatory. It alludes to the lemon-like aroma that emanates from its stalks. Yet, in the names it has been given, there's a tale of human experience. In its native land, it's known as *sera* in Sinhalese, meaning "spike", and *chera* in Malayalam, hinting at its blade-like appearance. Each name, in each language, is a chapter in the grand narrative of this herb.

Scent and Serenity: Aroma of Lemongrass

The moment lemongrass is crushed or boiled, it releases a citric symphony. The aroma is not merely about olfactory pleasure—it's a summon to a tropical haven. But this scent isn't just reminiscent of lemon. There's a grassy undertone, a subtle earthiness, and a hint of mint.

On the Palate: Tasting the Tropics

Beyond its fragrance, tasting lemongrass is an experience unto itself. The initial hit is unmistakably citric, but it's milder, more nuanced than its fruit counterpart. What follows is an orchestra of flavors—there's sweetness, there's the warmth of ginger, and a gentle aftertaste that lingers, reminiscent of roses kissed by morning dew.

Lemongrass: More Than Meets the Eye

While lemongrass graces many a kitchen and has endeared itself to countless palates, its significance isn't confined to the culinary. The plant, with its myriad uses, tells stories of traditions, of homes that smelled of its distinct aroma, and of ancient practices that revered it not just as a herb, but as a healer.

The Land of a Thousand Temples: Introducing Thailand

Against the rich tapestry of Southeast Asia lies a nation dotted with golden spires and bustling markets, with a river snaking its way through heartlands and echoing with chants from hidden temples: Thailand. Long before the tourists came flocking to its sun-kissed beaches, this was a realm of ancient kingdoms and rich traditions. From the early Ayutthaya kingdom to the mighty Sukhothai empire, Thailand's history is a mosaic of cultures, conflicts, and collaborations.

The Thai people, resilient and resourceful, with a renowned zest for life, have long had a harmonious bond with their land. Amidst the intricacies of their civilization, one constant remained – nature's role in their daily lives. And amongst nature's myriad offerings, lemongrass held a place of reverence.

Brewed Traditions: Lemongrass in the Thai Way of Life

In the labyrinthine streets of Bangkok or the tranquil villages nestled in the northern mountains, the invigorating aroma of lemongrass is as ubiquitous as the gentle smiles of the Thai people.

A Cup of Comfort: Lemongrass Tea and Thai Homes

Beyond its role in the celebrated Thai green curry or Tom Yum soup, lemongrass is an esteemed beverage. In traditional Thai households, the act of brewing lemongrass tea is almost ritualistic. The tall stalks, freshly plucked, are meticulously cleaned and chopped, then gently bruised to release their essence. When steeped in boiling water, they unfurl both their flavors and tales.

Though lemongrass tea can be enjoyed purely for its refreshing taste, for the Thai, it goes beyond sensory pleasure. The tea has been an age-old remedy, a grandmother's solution to a myriad of ailments - from the pesky flu to the agony of a bloated stomach.

The Spiritual Elixir: Lemongrass and Thai Temples
Thailand, with its deep-rooted Buddhist traditions, sees lemongrass not just as a culinary ingredient but also as a spiritual conduit. In the shadowy recesses of temples, the herb often finds its way into ceremonies and rituals.

For instance, during the Kathin ceremony, marking the end of the Buddhist Lent, offerings, including lemongrass, are made to monks. Its presence signifies purity, its aroma thought to cleanse spaces and beckon positive energies.

Modern Revelations: Health Benefits of Lemongrass Tea
The global palate has warmly embraced lemongrass, not merely for its zest but for the plethora of benefits lurking within its fibrous stalks.

Nature's Panacea
Rich in antioxidants, lemongrass tea is believed to combat free radicals, those cellular miscreants responsible for aging and cellular damage. Additionally, its anti-inflammatory properties make it a sought-after remedy for those grappling with arthritis or similar ailments.

For the stressed mind, a cup of this tea is akin to a gentle, aromatic embrace. With its mild sedative properties, it alleviates anxiety, ushering in a sense of calm.

Digestive Harmony

Long have the Thai people revered lemongrass for its role in digestion. Modern science concurs. The herb aids in regulating intestinal function and is often recommended for those battling indigestion or constipation.

Cautionary Tales: The Flip Side

Like all things, lemongrass tea, when consumed in excess, might not resonate well with all constitutions.

For some, especially those with a sensitive gut, the tea might exacerbate rather than alleviate digestive issues. Furthermore, those on medications for hypertension or diabetes should tread cautiously, for lemongrass can interfere with these medications.

Blending Notes: Lemongrass Meets its Herbal Companions

In the world of herbal infusions, blending is both an art and a science. Lemongrass, with its distinct profile, can either complement or conflict.

Synergistic Serenades

With chamomile, lemongrass finds a gentle companion. The blend is a lullaby in a cup. With peppermint, it's a rejuvenating duet, perfect for those midday slumps.

Brewed Dissonance

However, when paired with robust herbs like sage, the resultant brew might be too aggressive on the palate. Similarly, with valerian root, the combined sedative effects might be overwhelming for some.

The Echoes of Lemongrass in Thai Heritage

As we meander through the lanes of history, culture, and tradition, one truth becomes evident – lemongrass is not just a plant; it's a thread in the Thai cultural fabric. Whether in steaming cups held against the backdrop of setting suns, or in ancient temple rituals, it remains a testament to Thailand's enduring bond with nature and its bounties.

Lavender – Serenity's Floral Essence

In a gentle evening's embrace,
Amongst the whispering wind's grace,
Stands lavender, tall and serene,
Nature's tranquil, fragrant queen.

The Lavender Legacy: More than Just a Plant

The world over recognizes lavender. From the rolling hills of Provence to the rugged landscapes of the Mediterranean, this purple flower has not just flourished, but imprinted itself onto the very soul of cultures. Yet, to truly understand this botanical wonder, we must first delve into its very essence.

Lavender's Roots: Origins and Etymology

Botanically known as *Lavandula*, lavender belongs to the mint family, Lamiaceae. It's not just a single plant, but a genus comprising of over 30 known species. Its roots, metaphorically and botanically, reach deep into the sands of time, hinting at a Mediterranean origin.

The etymology of lavender is as poetic as its appearance. Derived from the Latin word "lavare," which means "to wash," it conjures images of Roman baths, where the flower often played a pivotal role. But the word also transcends the physical act of cleansing, hinting at a purification of the spirit, a sentiment resonating even today.

The Symphony of Senses: Aroma and Taste

Anyone who's ever been close to a lavender field will recount, often with a faraway look in their eyes, the almost magical aroma wafting through the air. It's a scent that lingers, both in the atmosphere and in the recesses of memory.

A Fragrance Unbound

Lavender's aroma is a complex tapestry of notes. There's the initial fresh floral burst, but it's underscored by subtle hints of mint and even rosemary. The scent is at once invigorating and calming, a duality that's perhaps at the heart of its widespread appeal.

For many, this aroma is not merely a sensory experience but a bridge to memories: summers spent in grandparents' gardens, the first trip to a quaint European village, or simply a moment of solace in a hectic day.

Tasting the Tinted Tisane

When brewed as a tea, lavender presents yet another facet of its intricate personality. The floral notes dominate, but there's a definite undertone of green, herbaceous freshness. Some even discern a slight camphoraceous taste, a gentle nod to its healing properties.

The taste of lavender tea is often described as a "gentle embrace." It doesn't jolt the palate like a robust black tea or enliven it like peppermint. Instead, it cradles it, offering warmth, comfort, and a subtle hint of the meadows it once called home.

The Roman World: A Civilizational Overview

Let's rewind the scroll of time, and find ourselves amidst the monumental structures, vast arenas, and bustling marketplaces of Ancient Rome. Here, an empire spanning three continents was bound not just by its legions and laws, but by the intertwining threads of culture and tradition.

Lavandula Romanus: Lavender's Place in the Heart of an Empire

The extensive trade routes of Rome brought many treasures from the far reaches of its dominions, but amongst these, it was often the simplest which held the most profound place in the daily lives of its citizens. Lavender, with its purifying Latin name, was such a treasure.

A Ritualistic Brew: The Conception of Lavender Tea

The Romans, for all their grandeur, held a deep appreciation for nature's offerings. It's no surprise then that the serene properties of lavender caught their discerning eye. While the concept of 'tea' as we understand it was alien to the ancient Romans, they indulged in a precursor: a brew of herbs and flowers, amongst which lavender stood out.

The steaming concoction was believed to be more than just a beverage. It was a ritual, a moment of reflection, and in some cases, a communion with the divine.

Sacred Scents and Spiritual Significance

In Rome's pantheon, multiple deities held dominion over different facets of life, and to appease or seek favors from these deities, rituals were essential. Lavender, with its tranquil aroma, was often a staple in these rites.

Vesta's Vigil

The goddess Vesta, the deity of home, hearth, and family, had her temple in the Roman Forum, where the eternal flame burned. Priests, the Vestal Virgins, maintained this flame, and it was here that lavender played its part. The dried sprigs, when thrown into the sacred fire, produced an aroma believed to purify the temple and invoke Vesta's blessings.

Somnus' Soothing Sips

Somnus, the deity of sleep, was another figure intricately linked to lavender. Before bedtime, many Romans drank a brew infused with lavender blossoms, believing it to be a potion that invoked Somnus' favor, ensuring a night of peaceful slumber.

Modern Echoes: Lavender's Enduring Health Benefits

From the apothecaries of Rome to the modern laboratories, lavender's reputation as a therapeutic wonder has endured. Numerous studies today testify to what the Romans instinctively knew. Lavender acts as a natural relaxant. In a world constantly on the edge, a simple cup of lavender tea serves as a bridge to tranquility.

Digestive Dynamo

The Romans often consumed rich foods, and lavender brews were their go-to post-meal. Today, we understand that lavender aids digestion, alleviating symptoms like bloating and gas.

Side Effects and Interactions

Every gift of nature comes with its own set of instructions, and lavender is no exception. While lavender is largely safe, overconsumption can lead to complications. Some individuals have reported headaches and constipation. It's crucial to heed one's body and find the optimal balance.

Interactions in the Cup

When blended with other herbal teas, lavender often plays well. However, when combined with sedative herbs like chamomile, the relaxing effects can be amplified, leading to drowsiness. On the other hand, when paired with invigorating teas like mint, lavender can offer a harmonious blend of rejuvenation and relaxation.

Lavender's Timeless Dance

To trace the journey of lavender is to journey through time itself. From ancient civilizations to modern high-end perfumeries, its presence is undeniable. Yet, at its heart, lavender remains a simple flower, swaying in the breeze, basking in the sun, and offering the world its scent, its flavor, and its very essence.

Dandelion - Nature's Gentle Detox

From field to cup, a journey begins,
Dandelion's taste, free of sins.
Wild essence, with a gentle grace,
Nature's touch, in every embrace.

The Humble Dandelion: Nature's Unassuming Marvel

At first glance, the dandelion might appear as nothing more than a common weed, attempting to claim its tiny kingdom within manicured lawns and fields. Yet, beneath its sunlit petals and delicate seeds, lies a story rich in history and brimming with potential.

The botanical name of dandelion, *Taraxacum officinale*, offers the first hint of its profound significance. Translated from its Greek origins, 'Taraxos' means 'disorder' and 'akos' signifies remedy. An elixir for disorder, as it were, waiting amidst the greens.

Origins & Etymology: Tracing the Roots of the Dandelion

The dandelion, a symbol of resilience, has ancient origins that crisscross continents. Fossils indicate its ancient presence in Eurasia, and its roots (both literal and historical) stretch deep into European and Asian traditions.

A Lion's Tooth

The word 'dandelion' rolls off the tongue with an elegant simplicity, but its etymology is a delightful blend of folklore and observation. Stemming from the French 'dent-de-lion', which translates to 'lion's tooth', the name references the jagged leaves of the plant, reminiscent of the fierce, sharp teeth of a lion.

A Symphony for the Senses: Dandelion's Aroma and Taste

To truly understand the appeal of dandelion tea, one must engage all the senses, letting the aroma and flavor tell their story.

A Scented Prelude

As the dandelion tea steeps, it releases a delicate aroma, a scent that is earthy with a hint of sweetness. It's a smell that evokes memories of dew-kissed mornings and the gentle rustle of leaves underfoot.

The First Sip

Upon tasting, the first note is a gentle bitterness, reminiscent of chicory. This is swiftly followed by a subtle sweetness, enveloping the palate in a harmonious blend. There's a mineral undertone, a connection to the deep-rooted nature of the plant. It's not just a flavor; it's an experience, a dialogue between the drinker and the earth from which the dandelion springs.

La Belle France: A Glimpse into a Historic Mélange

To understand the relationship the French have with the dandelion and its brew, it is paramount to first immerse oneself into the nuanced tapestry of French civilization. France, with its legacy stretching from the primal tribes of Gaul to the revolutionary spirit of Paris, is a land that marries tradition with evolution. It is amidst this mélange that the dandelion finds its cultural significance.

Dandelion's Place in French Herbology

The verdant fields of France are no strangers to the golden blooms of the dandelion. Its presence in the wild meadows of the French countryside is as emblematic as the lavender fields of Provence or the vineyards of Bordeaux.

A Medicinal Mainstay

Before it graced teacups, the dandelion was primarily recognized for its medicinal properties. Rooted deep in the annals of French herbalism, dandelions were prescribed by apothecaries for a plethora of ailments. Its diuretic nature earned it the French moniker 'pissenlit' (lit. 'wet the bed'), highlighting its usage in promoting renal health.

The French rural folks, with their profound understanding of their lands, were quick to recognize and incorporate the dandelion into their pharmacopeia. From concoctions for digestive wellness to tonics for liver ailments, the dandelion, unassuming as it might seem, played an important role in traditional French medicine.

Brewed in Tradition: Dandelion Tea in French Culture

To see dandelion only through a medicinal lens would be to ignore its subtle infiltration into the daily life and traditions of the French people. The act of foraging dandelions became more than a mere collection; it was a community activity. Sundays, after church, families would often head to fields, baskets in hand, in search of the finest dandelion greens. These outings were not just about the harvest but were infused with camaraderie, song, and shared meals.

The Culinary Delight

While dandelion tea is a subject of our exploration, it is worth noting the plant's culinary presence in French cuisine. The tender spring leaves often found their way into salads, seasoned lightly with vinaigrette, while roots were sometimes roasted as a coffee substitute.

Spirituality & Symbolism: Dandelion's Ethereal Bond

The French have an innate ability to find profound meaning in the simple things, and the dandelion was no exception. In the Christian majority nation, the dandelion, which blooms around the time of the Annunciation in late March, was often linked symbolically to the Virgin Mary. The golden hue of its petals was likened to the golden halo of the Madonna, symbolizing purity and resilience.

Modern Infusions: Health and Well-being

The significance of dandelion tea has only grown with time, evolving from its traditional uses to suit contemporary palates and needs. Modern science, in validating age-old wisdom, has revealed a spectrum of health benefits from dandelion consumption:

1. **Liver Health:** Dandelion tea acts as a detoxifier.

2. **Digestive Aid:** Its bitter compounds can stimulate digestive enzymes.

3. **Anti-inflammatory Properties:** It might help reduce inflammation.

4. **Skin Health:** Rich in antioxidants, it may combat free radicals leading to healthier skin.

Side-effects and Interactions

No herb, no matter its virtue, is without its cautions. Some individuals might experience allergies, especially those sensitive to plants like ragweed. Overconsumption might lead to digestive discomfort.

When blended with other teas, dandelion's robust profile might overshadow or enhance the characteristics of the accompanying herb. For instance, when paired with chamomile, another bitter herb, the resultant brew might become too potent for some.

The Resilient Legacy of Dandelion in France

From the sunlit meadows of Normandy to the patisseries of Paris, dandelion's mark on French civilization is indelible. It stands as a testament to the French spirit – resilient, vibrant, and forever evolving, yet rooted deep in history.

Nettle – The Ancient Brew of the Isles

Jagged leaves, aroma pure,
Nettle tea, the forest's allure.
From sting to soothing, its tale weaves,
Embracing senses, as it leaves.

Nettle's Proud Stature: More than Just a Weed

To the untrained eye, the nettle, with its serrated leaves and menacing hairs, may be dismissed as an inconsequential weed. But look closer, and one discovers a plant steeped in history, medicinal promise, and culinary prowess. Its botanical name, *Urtica dioica*, gives a nod to its burning sting – 'Urtica' coming from the Latin 'uro', meaning 'I burn'. It's a plant that demands respect and, once given, offers a cornucopia of benefits.

Origins: The Deep-rooted Legacy of Nettle

Nettle's history traces back to ancient times. Archaeologists have unearthed fabric remnants from Bronze Age settlements, indicating that our ancestors recognized nettle's potential for textile creation. In the moist and temperate climate of the British Isles, nettles thrived, becoming an integral part of the natural landscape.

Etymology: Words as Old as Time

The English word 'nettle' harks back to Old English, derived from 'netel'. Its Germanic roots can be traced to the word 'nazza', and even further back, to the Proto-Indo-European base 'ned' – a testament to its ancient presence in human civilization.

A Whiff of Earth: The Aroma of Nettle Tea

There's an earthiness to nettle tea, reminiscent of the rain-soaked soils of England's vast meadows. The aroma, both grounding and invigorating, evokes images of ancient Druid rituals, of stone circles cloaked in morning mist, and of endless green expanses under the ever-changing English sky. This isn't a scent that shouts but whispers, telling tales of old.

Tasting Time: Sip by Ancient Sip

The taste profile of nettle tea mirrors its aroma but with added layers. There's a gentle sweetness, a touch of the salty sea breeze, and a distant, almost elusive bitterness – like the fleeting English summers. This isn't a beverage that requires an acquired taste; it's one that asks you to remember, to hark back to a time when man and nature were intertwined.

The English Tapestry: Threads of History and Landscape

The story of England is one of resilience, innovation, and profound connection to the land. From the Druids who once worshipped among the ancient stones of Stonehenge, through the fervor of the Reformation, to the smog-filled alleys of Industrial Revolution-era London, England has consistently been a land of contrasts. Yet, the natural world, with its mists, moors, and meadows, has always held a special place in the English soul.

Brewed from the Earth: Nettle's Role in English Heritage

Hidden among the lore of knights and castles, nettle tea finds its niche. While it might not boast the legendary status of Excalibur or the Round Table, it remains a fixture in the story of the English people.

For the denizens of Medieval England, particularly in rural locales, the common nettle was far more than a stinging pest. It was a vital component of their pharmacopeia, a source of nourishment, and, in the form of tea, a comforting draught in times both good and harsh.

A Spiritual Brew? The Mystical Side of Nettle Tea

As with many natural remedies, the line between the physical and spiritual was often blurred in ancient and medieval beliefs. To understand nettle tea's place in this tapestry, we must turn our gaze to the old practices and beliefs.

The Druids, though more associated with ancient Celtic practices, left an indelible mark on English spiritual traditions. Plants were not just medicinal or food; they were bridges to the divine, each with its spirit or essence. While the oak was their tree of reverence, other plants like the nettle had their roles in rituals and rites.

Certain old wives' tales suggest that nettles had protective qualities. A brew of nettle tea was believed to guard one against malevolent spirits and spells. In an age where the supernatural was as real as the air one breathed, such protective measures, even in the form of a simple tea, were invaluable.

Modern Times: The Resurgence of Nettle Tea

As the centuries progressed, the onslaught of the Industrial Revolution and the rise of modern medicine saw many turn away from the traditional remedies of their forebears. Yet, in the latter half of the 20th century, a revival began. A renewed interest in organic living, combined with a desire to reconnect with ancestral practices, led many back to the arms of nettle tea.

Today, you'd find nettle tea gracing the shelves of organic stores across England, hailed for its myriad health benefits. It's no longer just a rustic brew; it's a beverage for the health-conscious modern individual.

Nettle's Generous Offering: Health Benefits and Modern Uses

The modern Englishman or woman turns to nettle tea not just for its taste but for its health promises:

- **Detoxification:** Nettle tea is renowned for its diuretic properties, aiding in the elimination of toxins.

- **Anti-inflammatory:** Those suffering from joint pains or arthritis might find relief in this age-old beverage.

- **Digestive Aid:** It has been suggested that nettle tea can alleviate issues like bloating, gas, and even constipation.

- **Skin and Hair:** Rich in antioxidants and beneficial compounds, nettle tea is believed to promote skin and hair health.

Side Effects and Interactions

While nettle tea is generally safe for consumption, like all things, it should be enjoyed in moderation. Overconsumption can lead to stomach issues or exacerbate kidney problems due to its diuretic nature.

Pregnant or breastfeeding women are often advised to avoid nettle tea, given the lack of comprehensive studies on its effects during these stages.

Moreover, those on medications, particularly diuretics or blood pressure drugs, should consult with their healthcare provider before adding nettle tea to their regimen.

A Symphony of Flavors: Nettle in Blends

Nettle tea, with its earthy and mildly herbaceous flavor, offers a versatile base for blends. When combined with other herbal teas, the results can be both delightful and beneficial.

- **Nettle and Peppermint:** For a refreshing twist, peppermint complements nettle's earthiness, providing a cooling aftertaste.

- **Nettle and Chamomile:** This blend promises a calming experience, perfect for unwinding after a long day.

- **Nettle and Rosehip:** For an added dose of Vitamin C and a subtle fruity note, rosehip proves an excellent companion to nettle.

In Conclusion: Nettle Tea - England's Green Gold

From the verdant countryside to the bustling streets of London, nettle tea stands as a testament to England's enduring bond with its natural heritage. It's a story of resilience, a tale of a humble plant that has woven itself into the fabric of English history.

Yarrow – The Ancient Healer

Feathered leaves, blooms so white,
Yarrow stands, bathed in light.
Sentinel of fields, guardian of lore,
Beauty and power, forevermore.

From Petals to Cup: The Yarrow Plant

Delicacy in strength – that is the yarrow. *Achillea millefolium*, its scientific nomenclature, hints at a warrior's legacy. With feathery leaves and clusters of tiny white to pink flowers, this perennial seems far removed from the brutalities of battlefields. Yet, as history unveils, yarrow's soft appearance belies its robust nature and the profound impact it has had on various civilizations.

Yarrow is a cosmopolitan plant, spanning across the temperate regions of the Northern Hemisphere. Its preferred residences are those of meadows, grasslands, and even the disturbed soils of roadsides and fields.

Origins and Etymology: Yarrow's Linguistic Journey

The word 'yarrow' is believed to be of Germanic origin, derived from the Old High German *garwa*, meaning 'prepare' or 'gear'. It's a name that subtly nods to the plant's utility and readiness.

But it's the Latin name, *Achillea millefolium*, that tells a more vivid story. The genus *Achillea* references the legendary Greek hero Achilles, and 'millefolium', translating to 'thousand leaves', speaks of its finely divided, fern-like foliage.

An Olfactory and Gustatory Experience: Yarrow's Aroma and Taste

To understand yarrow, one must engage with it sensorially. Crush a yarrow leaf between fingers, and it releases a distinct aroma. Herbal with a touch of camphor, there's an echo of ancient woods and whispered secrets in its scent. It's an evocative fragrance, bridging the modern world with echoes from eons past.

Steeped as a tea, yarrow transforms. The camphorous note softens, making way for a mildly astringent, slightly bitter flavor with an undertone of sweetness. It's a taste that reminds one of green meadows after a light spring rain, refreshing and subtly invigorating.

The History in its Roots

Before it was a tea, yarrow was a tool. Early humans, recognizing its resilient nature, used it for a variety of purposes. Archaeological excavations across Europe, particularly at burial sites, have uncovered traces of yarrow pollen, hinting at its spiritual or medicinal significance even in prehistoric times.

Evidence even suggests that Neanderthals, in what is now modern-day Iraq, might have used yarrow as a part of their medicinal toolkit. Such discoveries indicate that our connection with this humble plant predates even the earliest civilizations, stretching back to our prehistoric ancestors.

The Greek Landscape: Where Ideas and Civilizations Flourished

The Mediterranean has always been a melting pot, a nexus of cultures, each contributing their own flavor to a vibrant tapestry. Dominating this ancient landscape was the civilization of the Greeks – a people known for their philosophers, warriors, and artists. With the Aegean Sea lapping at its shores and the formidable Mount Olympus piercing the horizon, Greece was a land of contrasts – as much in its topography as in its ideas.

Yarrow's Grecian Tale: Beyond Achilles

While the etymology of yarrow – *Achillea millefolium* – hearkens back to the warrior Achilles, this plant's connection with Ancient Greece is more intricate than mere namesakes. As often is the case with the Greeks, it intertwines the practical with the poetic, the mythic with the mundane.

Herbal Medicine and the Greek Physicians

The Greeks, with their scientific curiosity and systematic approach, were pioneers in herbal medicine. Thinkers like Hippocrates and Dioscorides penned extensive texts detailing the medicinal properties of plants. Yarrow, with its myriad benefits, found its due mention.

In his pharmacopeia, Dioscorides spoke of yarrow's ability to staunch wounds, a property that likely contributed to its association with Achilles, the warrior who was said to have used it on the battlefield. The ancients recognized yarrow's capacity to alleviate fevers, aid digestion, and as a remedy for various women's ailments.

Achilles and the Yarrow Connection

In Greek mythology, Achilles is best known as the legendary warrior of the Trojan War, a key character in Homer's "Iliad." His strength, skill, and combat prowess were unparalleled, except for one vulnerable point: his heel, the so-called "Achilles' heel."

As the myth goes, Achilles was taught the healing properties of yarrow by his tutor Chiron, the centaur. Chiron was a wise and benevolent figure known for his vast knowledge in medicine and herbs. Under his guidance, Achilles learned to use yarrow to treat and staunch the wounds of his soldiers during the Trojan War. The herb's astringent properties helped in stopping the bleeding and promoting healing.

While the "Iliad" itself doesn't delve into detailed herbology, later interpretations and historical accounts picked up on this association, linking the warrior and the plant. Over time, yarrow became known as an essential herb for wound healing, thanks in part to this mythological endorsement.

In Rituals and Spirituality

The Greeks didn't merely perceive plants in utilitarian terms. The land of Dionysian mysteries and Orphic hymns lent a spiritual hue to much of its flora. Yarrow, with its delicate flowers and resilience, became a symbol of protection. It was not uncommon to find it hanging at doorways or woven into bridal bouquets, acting as a talisman against malevolent forces.

Yarrow in Delphic Divinations

Delphi, the navel of the ancient world, was a hub of spiritual and prophetic activities. Here, yarrow took on another role – as an instrument of divination. Stalks of yarrow, dried and inscribed with symbols, were cast onto sacred grounds to glean insights into the future or seek answers to perplexing questions.

From Antiquity to Modernity: Yarrow's Timeless Benefits

Fast forward a few millennia, and yarrow's reputation as a healer remains unscathed. Modern science, with its penchant for probing and dissecting, has come to echo what the ancients instinctively knew.

A Treasure Trove of Health Benefits

Today, yarrow tea, with its gentle bitterness, is sought not just for its taste but for its therapeutic benefits. Studies have revealed its potential in:

1. **Digestive Health**: Just as Dioscorides wrote, yarrow aids digestion. Its bitter compounds stimulate bile production, aiding in the breakdown of fats.

2. **Anti-inflammatory Properties**: The tea is known to possess anti-inflammatory agents, beneficial in conditions like arthritis or swelling.

3. **Cardiovascular Support**: Yarrow has been shown to improve circulation, making it beneficial for heart health.

Possible Side Effects

While yarrow's accolades are many, like all potent herbs, it comes with its cautions. Consumed in moderate amounts, yarrow tea is safe for most people. However, excessive consumption might lead to:

- Photosensitivity in some individuals.

- Allergic reactions, especially in those allergic to plants in the Asteraceae family.

- Possible interactions with blood pressure and blood-thinning medications.

When Yarrow Meets Other Herbs: A Symphony of Interactions

Herbal teas often sing louder in blends. Yarrow, with its unique profile, can either complement or clash, depending on its partner.

1. **Yarrow and Chamomile**: Both being from the Asteraceae family, they share certain therapeutic compounds. Together, they can amplify relaxation and digestive benefits.

2. **Yarrow and Mint**: Mint's coolness can offset yarrow's bitterness, creating a balanced brew.

3. **Yarrow and St. John's Wort**: This combination should be approached with caution. Both herbs, while beneficial on their own, can potentiate each other's side effects.

In Reflection: Yarrow's Persistent Whisper

From the sun-kissed landscapes of Ancient Greece to the scientific laboratories of today, yarrow's narrative remains unwavering. It stands as a testament to nature's unyielding potency and mankind's perpetual quest for understanding. The delicate yarrow, with its feathery leaves and whispers of legends, continues to beckon – offering wellness, wisdom, and a window into our shared past.

Licorice Root - Nature's Sweetened Solace

Earthy whispers, a hint of sweet,
Licorice aroma, a fragrant treat.
Memories of ancient, and tales untold,
Unfurling slowly, bold and old.

The Rooted Legacy

It's easy to walk through life, letting everyday treasures fade into the unnoticed background. Like the subtle but present influence of an old painting in a room, licorice root, often understated, has woven its story through millennia, offering its gifts generously to all who care to recognize them.

Origins: Beneath Earth's Crust

Licorice root, or *Glycyrrhiza glabra*, is no newcomer to the herbal stage. Its history is as deep and intertwined as the root system from which it comes. Native to parts of Asia and southern Europe, licorice's verdant leaves and purple to pale whitish-blue flowers give little hint to the treasure that lies beneath the surface. For below the soil, the plant hides its most precious resource: long, woody roots with a sweet, rich flavor.

The name *Glycyrrhiza* is a union of ancient appreciation, derived from the Greek words "glykys," meaning sweet, and "rhiza," meaning root. Indeed, the root's sweetness is almost deceptive, being fifty times sweeter than sugar. But its sweetness isn't just about flavor; it's a reflection of the root's rich history and multifaceted applications.

A Symphony of Senses: Aroma and Taste

Even before one sips a cup of licorice tea, the aroma makes a gentle, persuasive introduction. It's a scent that recalls ancient marketplaces, a melding of woody notes with a hint of sweetness, promising a journey not just for the taste buds but for the soul.

And when one finally tastes it, it is a crescendo. First, there's the unmistakable sweetness, almost molasses-like, thick and enveloping. But then, a more complex profile emerges—woody, earthy, with a faint hint of anise. It's a taste that recalls both its ancient uses as a sweetener and its medicinal properties, a bridge between pleasure and function.

The Assyrians: Pillars of the Ancient World

Perched atop the cradle of civilization, the Assyrians emerged as a powerful empire, their dominion stretching from modern-day Iraq to parts of Turkey, Syria, and Iran. Their robust city-states, grandeur-filled art, and sophisticated bureaucracy established them as one of the major players of the Mesopotamian narrative. Yet, amid the tales of their military might and architectural prowess, lie subtle traces of their intimate relationship with nature. And within this tapestry of flora and fauna, licorice root held its special corner.

Licorice: The Assyrian Nectar

The use of licorice in Assyrian culture can be traced through the numerous clay tablets that have survived the ravages of time. These inscriptions, primarily serving as medical texts, suggest that licorice was highly valued for its medicinal properties.

Medicinal Elixirs: Healing in Every Sip

The Assyrians, much like their Mesopotamian counterparts, believed in the synergy of mind, body, and spirit. Illnesses were often perceived as the displeasure of gods or the result of evil spirits. Healing, therefore, was a blend of the spiritual and the physical.

Licorice was frequently employed as a remedial agent in this process. The root was recognized for its demulcent properties, which means it soothed and protected irritated mucous membranes. For the Assyrians, this translated to a potent remedy for stomach ailments, respiratory troubles, and even for the discomforts of the liver.

In the ancient city of Ashur, a major hub of trade, licorice concoctions were likely dispensed in the marketplaces by Assyrian healers, standing next to stalls of shimmering textiles and handcrafted jewelry. Here, licorice wasn't just a drink; it was a curative, a bridge between the ethereal and the tangible.

Cultural Resonance: More Than Just a Beverage

Licorice's significance wasn't limited to its medicinal properties. Its sweetness made it a desired ingredient in the royal kitchens, offering a refined palate for the elite. The root, with its rich, earthy sweetness, was often paired with other aromatic spices like cardamom and cinnamon to produce beverages fit for kings.

But there's more. Assyrian rituals, infused with the rich cadence of hymns, involved offerings to the deities. Amid the ceremonial foods, licorice-infused concoctions likely found their place as an offering to appease the gods, drawing them closer to the world of mortals.

The Modern Elixir: Healing in the Contemporary

Time, as it is wont to, moved ahead, but licorice root's influence remained undiminished. Today, this ancient remedy has been repackaged into modern wellness. Its therapeutic properties are recognized worldwide, finding their way into teas, syrups, and even pharmaceutical preparations.

Research underscores its anti-inflammatory and immune-boosting properties, providing relief from gastrointestinal problems and acting as a potent antioxidant. The sweet root also holds potential in the regulation of cortisol, the body's stress hormone, hinting at its role in managing modern-day stress and anxiety.

A Word of Caution: The Two Edges of the Blade

Every coin has two sides, and licorice is no exception. While it possesses a plethora of health benefits, its overconsumption can lead to complications. Glycyrrhizin, the primary active component, when consumed in large amounts, can cause a decrease in potassium levels in the body. This, in turn, can lead to high blood pressure, edema, and even heart-related issues.

It's a gentle reminder that even the most potent remedies from nature need to be respected and consumed in moderation.

Interactions with Herbal Siblings

In the world of herbal blends, licorice often finds itself intertwined with other herbs, enhancing flavors and potentiating therapeutic effects. However, it's crucial to understand its interactions.

When blended with peppermint, for instance, the concoction can provide an amplified relief from digestive troubles. Paired with echinacea, it might boost immune responses. But caution must be exercised when mixing with other herbs that influence potassium levels or blood pressure. The sweet symphony of licorice, while melodious, must be orchestrated with care.

The Timeless Dance

The journey of licorice, from the ancient city-state of Ashur to the modern teacups, is a testament to the timeless bond between humans and nature. For the Assyrians, licorice wasn't just a plant; it was a slice of the divine, a thread connecting them to the cosmos. Today, as we sip our licorice teas, we partake in that ancient ritual, that eternal dance between humanity and the universe.

Elderflower – The Immune Boosting Bloom

Delicate breezes, hints of spring,
Elderflower's scent, on dove's wing.
A fragrance gentle, pure, and light,
Like moonlit dreams, soft and bright.

The Elder Tree: A Chronicle of Ages

As ancient as the wind that rustles through its leaves, the Elder tree stands as a sentinel to history, its gnarled branches bearing testament to countless sunrises and sunsets. The tree, scientifically known as *Sambucus*, belongs to a genus of flowering plants in the family Adoxaceae. Its blossoms, delicate and fragrant, have captivated the senses of those who wandered the woods for millennia.

Though the Elder tree generously bears both flowers and berries, it is the flowers, those intricate clusters of creamy white, that have silently brewed a legacy in the annals of herbal tea. Their ephemeral nature, appearing for but a fleeting moment in the late spring, only adds to their allure.

Etymology: Echoes from a Time Long Past

The term 'elder' traces its lineage back to the Old English word 'ellærn'. Even further back, the Proto-Germanic term '*aluz*', which denotes the tree, hints at an even older origin. The journey of a name, much like a river, meanders through cultures and epochs, collecting stories and sentiments. The very act of sipping Elderflower tea becomes a communion with these ancient tongues.

The Aroma: Nature's Symphony

It is said that to truly understand the soul of the Elderflower, one must first lose oneself in its aroma. This is not the heady perfume of roses or the intoxicating scent of jasmine. Instead, Elderflower whispers its presence, a delicate fragrance reminiscent of honeyed meadows and the gentle touch of spring's first light. It's an olfactory tapestry where notes of muscat grape intertwine with subtle hints of fresh-cut grass.

A Taste of Timelessness

If its aroma is a whisper, the taste of Elderflower tea is a gentle conversation. Upon the first sip, the palate is introduced to a soft sweetness, almost ethereal in its quality. This is swiftly followed by a light, citrusy undertone, reminiscent of the lemon groves under the Mediterranean sun. Yet, underneath it all lies a depth, an earthiness that grounds the drinker, a reminder that this brew has its roots in the very heart of nature.

Origins: The Dance of Geology and Botany

While it's tempting to think of the Elder tree as a static entity, its history is one of migration and adaptation. Originally native to Europe, it has since whispered its way across the continents, finding homes in Asia and even North Africa. Over time, various species of the tree have evolved, each adapting to its specific environment, yet all bearing the signature clusters of fragrant blossoms.

It is believed that the Elder tree thrived in the post-glacial period, capitalizing on the newly fertile soils and rapidly colonizing the European landscape. This adaptability, combined with its inherent resilience, ensured that the Elder became a mainstay in ancient European groves.

The Celts: A Tapestry of Tribes and Traditions

Before we tread upon the ancient groves where Elderflowers bloomed and were tenderly plucked by Celtic hands, it's paramount to know those hands and the hearts that guided them. The Celts, an assortment of tribes spread across Europe, have long evoked images of fierce warriors with blue-painted faces and intricate tattoos. Yet, to pigeonhole them solely into this silhouette is to do them an injustice.

Originating from Central Europe around 1200 B.C., the Celts swiftly expanded in every direction, each tribe carrying with it unique traditions, deities, and practices. Theirs was not the civilization of grand empires or colossal stone structures; instead, the Celts etched their legacy upon the landscape, upon art, and most vitally, upon the European psyche.

The Sacred Grove: Nature's Altar

For the Celts, nature wasn't just a backdrop to life; it was life. Their spiritual practices, often grouped under the umbrella term 'Druidism', were intrinsically tied to the land. The Oak was venerated, rivers were considered divine, and the groves were sacred spaces, where the veil between the mortal realm and the otherworld was thin.

It was in these groves that the Elder tree often found a home. To the Celts, trees were not mere vegetation; they were entities, each with its spirit, its energy, and its place in the cosmic dance.

Elderflower in Celtic Brews: More than Just a Beverage

Elderflower's entrance into the Celtic world wasn't heralded with grand ceremonies or written records. Instead, its journey was organic, much like the tree itself. But to discern how Elderflower might have been consumed by the Celts, one has to think beyond the paradigm of modern tea.

While the exact recipes and methods remain lost to time, it's likely that Elderflowers, given their aromatic properties, found their way into fermented drinks. Meads or ales infused with herbs and flowers were not uncommon. The addition of Elderflower not only added a delicate flavor but also, perhaps, a touch of the divine.

A Symbol of Protection and Healing

In the tapestry of Celtic spirituality, where every tree held significance, the Elder was often seen as a protector. Its presence near a dwelling was believed to ward off malevolent spirits. More than just spiritual, this protective aura extended to the physical realm.

The Celts, with their deep understanding of the natural world, recognized the medicinal properties of the plants around them. Elderflower's diaphoretic nature, its ability to induce sweating, made it valuable in treating fevers and other maladies.

Modern Embrace: From Ancient Groves to Contemporary Cups

As centuries turned and the world transformed, the Elderflower's charm didn't wane. Today, it finds itself in kitchens and cafes, not just in its native Europe, but across the globe. But why this undying allure?

Apart from its ethereal taste, Elderflower tea is a treasure trove of health benefits. Rich in antioxidants, it's a modern-day elixir for skin health, potentially aiding in reducing the signs of aging and warding off damage from free radicals. The age-old belief in its ability to combat colds and flu finds validation in its antiviral properties.

Yet, like all good things, moderation is key. Excessive consumption can lead to digestive issues or exacerbate allergies in susceptible individuals.

Blends and Companions: The Alchemy of Herbs

The world of herbal teas is not one of isolation but of interaction. When Elderflower meets another herb in a brew, magic happens. Take, for instance, the pairing of Elderflower with chamomile, another ancient favorite. While Elderflower brings its light, floral notes, chamomile contributes its calming properties, creating a blend that's both flavorful and therapeutic.

However, blending isn't mere guesswork. It requires an understanding of each herb's properties to ensure that they enhance rather than negate each other. For someone with low blood pressure, a blend of Elderflower, known to be hypotensive, with another herb possessing similar properties might not be advisable.

Conclusion: A Legacy in Blossoms

As we trace our fingers over the tapestry of time, feeling the intricate patterns of civilizations, beliefs, and traditions, the Elderflower stands out, not because of its grandeur but because of its humility. To the Celts, it was a bridge between the realms, a symbol of protection, and a source of sustenance. In our modern world, it's a sip of serenity, a gulp of the past, and a toast to the timeless dance of nature and culture.

Rosehip - A Brew from the Heart of Thorns

A breath of petals, wild and free,
Rosehip's scent, nature's decree.
Whispering tales of ancient bloom,
Filling hearts, dispelling gloom.

From Bloom to Berry: The Life of Rosehip

While roses are celebrated, serenaded, and even venerated, their hips - the round fruit that appears post the bloom - often remain overlooked. But delve deeper, and you'll uncover a world as rich, if not richer, than the blossoms themselves.

The term 'hip' in rosehip is derived from the Old English 'hēope' and the Old High German 'hiafi', both alluding to the rose fruit. The rose plant, in its multitude of species, paints a picture that's both wild and cultivated, ancient and ever-renewing.

Origins and Travels

Rosehips aren't the offspring of the tender, grafted roses that grace ornate gardens. They hail from the wild roses, the dog roses (*Rosa canina*), the ones that stand unpruned, unhindered, bearing witness to winds, rains, and the dance of time. These wild roses are believed to be native to Europe, western Asia, and northwest Africa.

Yet, the story of rosehips isn't confined to its native lands. Like the petals that ride the winds, the tale of rosehips is one of travels and transformations. Carried by traders, travelers, birds, and breezes, the wild rose and its fruit have found homes in distant lands, from the Americas to the far reaches of Asia.

The Aroma: Subtle Whispers of Forests and Fields

To describe the aroma of rosehip tea is to pen a love letter to the wilderness. It doesn't besiege the senses like the intense fragrance of a blooming rose. Instead, it beckons you gently, subtly. There's a hint of tartness, reminiscent of crab apples, a distant cousin of roses. This is intertwined with a woody undertone, a whisper from the forests where wild roses often thrive.

Tasting the Wild

The first sip of rosehip tea might catch one off guard, especially if they're expecting the floral symphony of rose petals. This isn't a delicate brew; it's forthright but nuanced. There's an initial tanginess, akin to a mild citrus fruit, followed by a warmth that hints at spices and earth. It's the taste of nature, unadulterated.

Etymology: A Linguistic Voyage

The journey of a word often mirrors the journey of the entity it represents. 'Rosehip' is no different. The term 'rose' can be traced back to Latin 'rosa', which itself might have roots in the ancient Iranian *wrda*. When the wild rose traveled, so did its name, undergoing subtle changes, adapting, yet retaining its core.

'Hip', as previously mentioned, has Germanic origins, subtly pointing towards the northern trysts of the wild rose, where it brushed against snow and bore fruit even in the cold embrace of winter.

The Vikings: Masters of Sea and Soil

At the cusp of the eighth century, from the rugged landscapes of Scandinavia, emerged a seafaring people whose name would echo through the annals of history: the Vikings. Often pictured as horned-helmet marauders, their narrative is both richer and more intricate than popular culture often depicts.

The Vikings weren't just raiders; they were traders, settlers, and explorers, their longships cutting through icy waters to discover, among other lands, what we now know as Greenland and Newfoundland. In their homelands, they farmed and fished, resilient against the biting northern cold, always seeking resources to sustain and heal themselves.

Rosehips in the Viking Pantry

In the far north, where winters were fierce and the ground often resisted, the Vikings found an ally in the wild dog rose. This hardy shrub, native to Europe but most suited to the northern climes, produced the small, red fruit known as rosehips. But did these formidable warriors truly pay heed to this modest berry?

There is archaeological evidence to suggest that the Vikings, particularly in settled communities, were adept at foraging. Amid the findings of seeds, grains, and bones, rosehips too make their modest appearance, indicating that these fruits were consumed.

A Tea for the Hardened Warrior

Rosehips, rich in Vitamin C, would have been invaluable in the colder regions where fresh produce was scant during the winters. While there isn't direct evidence of the Vikings brewing rosehip tea, the act of boiling berries and herbs to extract their essence was known in the medieval world.

Imagine, if you will, a Viking settler, weary from a day's toil, sipping on a hot brew made from boiled rosehips. The tangy taste, the warmth seeping into the bones, reinvigorating the spirit, readying him for the next day's endeavors.

Spiritual Significance: Nature's Gifts

The Vikings, despite their often ferocious reputation, had a deep spiritual connection to the land and its produce. Their pantheon, with gods like Freyr and Freyja, celebrated fertility and harvests. While the rosehip doesn't make a prominent appearance in their myths, it's not hard to see it as one of nature's gifts, a token from the gods for survival.

To the Vikings, every element of nature, every tree, berry, or herb had a spirit. Consuming these was not just about physical sustenance but also about imbibing their essence, their strength.

Rosehip Tea: The Modern Elixir

Fast forward a millennium and rosehip tea has transcended its Viking past to become a cherished brew worldwide. The reasons aren't just gustatory but also therapeutic.

Rich in Vitamin C, rosehip tea is touted for its immune-boosting properties. Moreover, the presence of polyphenols, flavonoids, and ellagic acid lends it anti-inflammatory and antioxidant characteristics. Modern studies suggest that regular consumption can aid in reducing symptoms of osteoarthritis, enhancing skin health, and possibly even supporting heart health.

A Word of Caution

Like all good things, rosehip tea too must be consumed in moderation. Excessive intake may lead to certain side effects. Some individuals might experience nausea, stomach cramps, or headaches. Given its high Vitamin C content, overconsumption can lead to symptoms like insomnia or increased thirst.

Furthermore, rosehip may act as a diuretic. Those with kidney issues or those taking diuretic medications should approach with caution and preferably under guidance from a health professional.

The Alchemy of Blends: Rosehip's Dance with Other Herbs

Rosehip's tangy taste lends itself beautifully to blends. Often, it's mixed with hibiscus, enhancing the tartness and the vibrant red hue of the brew. But beyond taste, how do these herbs interact?

Hibiscus and rosehip together create a Vitamin C powerhouse, making the blend particularly beneficial during cold and flu seasons. Another common companion is chamomile, the apple-like aroma of which complements rosehip's tanginess. This blend, while flavorful, also combines rosehip's antioxidants with chamomile's calming properties.

Mint, with its cooling essence, often dances with the warmth of rosehip, creating a brew that's refreshing and rejuvenating at once. However, those with heartburn or acid reflux issues might want to approach this blend with caution.

From Viking Shores to Modern Mugs
The journey of the rosehip, from the wild landscapes of Scandinavia to teacups worldwide, is emblematic of the enduring human spirit, of resilience, discovery, and adaptation. The Vikings, in their quests for survival and dominance, unknowingly championed a berry that would stand the test of time, its legacy steeped in every brew, its history sipped and savored.

Fennel – Digestion's Fragrant Aid

A scent of anise, sweet and clear,
Fennel's whisper, drawing near.
Fragrance of gardens, fresh and green,
Inviting moments of serenity unseen.

Introducing Foeniculum vulgare: The Latin Vestige

The scientific name of fennel, *Foeniculum vulgare*, is a whisper, a soft murmur that speaks of antiquity and Latin etymology. Derived from the Latin word 'foenum', meaning hay, this nomenclature pays homage to its aromatic similarity to the freshly harvested grasses that fed the livestock of ancient civilizations.

To say that the name is a vestige is an understatement. In it lies an echo of a time when language was not merely a means of communication but a bridge that connected humans to nature, encapsulating their observations, their wonder, their relationships with the flora that surrounded them.

Fennel: A Glimpse at Its Origins

Sprouting wild across the shores of the Mediterranean, fennel's tale is as old as civilization itself. It's a story of survival, thriving in sandy soils and rocky outcrops, its roots burrowing deep to quench its thirst from underground streams, its feathery fronds playing with the salty sea breezes.

Its journey from the wild landscapes of its birth to gardens and farms is intertwined with human discovery. As the ancients realized its culinary and medicinal prowess, fennel became a cherished plant, cultivated with care, traded with passion, and consumed with reverence.

A Scented Symphony: The Aroma and Palate of Fennel

Approaching a fennel plant, even before your fingers touch its green tendrils, you are greeted by a fragrance. It's subtle yet assertive, reminiscent of aniseed but softer, more earthy. The scent is an invitation, beckoning one closer, hinting at the flavor held within.

When brewed into a tea, fennel releases its volatile oils, the water turning a light golden, the aroma filling the room like a scented symphony. On the palate, it is softly sweet, with a licorice-like undertone, a hint of earthiness grounding the experience. The finish is clean, leaving behind a lingering warmth, a reminder of its Mediterranean origins.

Fennel's Gift to Humanity

If one were to walk the annals of time, fennel would emerge as a constant companion to humanity. A wild herb that so captured the ancient imagination that it was tamed, cultivated, and woven into the very fabric of their daily lives. Its name, its scent, its taste, are not mere sensory experiences. They are historical markers, each telling a tale, each a testament to our age-old relationship with the world around us.

Byzantium: A Lustrous Civilization Unfolds

At the crossroads of Europe and Asia, where the Golden Horn kisses the Bosphorus, rose a civilization that would stand as an emblem of endurance and magnificence for over a millennium – the Byzantine Empire. More than just a continuation of the Roman legacy, the Byzantines intricately wove their Greco-Roman heritage with the richness of the orient, creating a tapestry luminous with art, culture, and tradition. Against this backdrop, we uncover the golden thread of fennel tea, tracing its journey through the intricate patterns of Byzantine life.

Bridging Gastronomy and Healing: Fennel's Dual Role in Byzantium

The Physician's Elixirs

Byzantine medicine, while carrying forward the traditions of Hippocrates and Galen, was also influenced by the Persians, Syriacs, and Arabs. Fennel, already known to the ancients for its remedial properties, found a venerated place in the Byzantine apothecary.

Physicians, carrying on the Hellenic traditions, believed in the balance of humors. Fennel, with its warming properties, was considered a balancer for cold and wet humors. It was prescribed for various respiratory ailments, particularly coughs. The seeds, crushed and brewed, would release oils known to ease bronchial passages.

Further, fennel's diuretic properties were recognized, making it a prescribed remedy for urinary issues. The sweet-tasting herb also served as a natural breath freshener, a subtle yet significant tool in the Byzantine world known for its elaborate social etiquettes.

The Byzantine Table

While it played a medicinal role, fennel was no stranger to the Byzantine kitchen. It graced the tables of both the elite and the commoner, its feathery fronds and crunchy bulbs accompanying various dishes, from fresh salads to hearty stews. The seeds, often toasted, lent their warm flavor to bread and pastries.

Symbolism: More than Just a Herb

To the Byzantines, every element had its place in the spiritual and cultural panorama. Fennel, with its hardy nature and fragrant blooms, became a symbol of strength and valor. Its towering stalks, reaching for the heavens, were seen as a metaphor for spiritual aspiration.

It wasn't uncommon for fennel fronds to be used during religious ceremonies, their fragrant wisps believed to purify the air, bridging the mundane with the divine.

Echoes in Modern Times: Health and Harmony

Fennel's popularity has not waned with the sands of time. Today, its benefits, both as a culinary herb and medicinal plant, resonate with a global audience.

Nutritional and Health Powerhouse

Modern science backs many of the health claims that the Byzantine physicians believed. Rich in dietary fiber, vitamin C, calcium, magnesium, and iron, fennel promotes heart health, aids digestion, and is anti-inflammatory. Its anethole compound is recognized for its potential anti-cancer properties.

Furthermore, the calming effects of fennel tea on the digestive system are widely acknowledged. It serves as a remedy for bloating, gas, and indigestion, a soothing balm for the agitated gut.

Cautionary Tales: Not All Roses

However, like all potent herbs, fennel comes with its cautions. Consumed in excess, it might lead to photodermatitis in some individuals. Furthermore, being a potent diuretic, excessive consumption could lead to dehydration.

Pregnant and nursing mothers, as well as individuals with estrogen-sensitive conditions, should exercise caution, as fennel has estrogen-like properties.

The Art of Blending: Fennel's Dance with Other Herbs

Fennel, with its sweet undertones, plays well with other herbs. Blended with peppermint, it aids digestion; with chamomile, it promotes calmness. However, when blending, one must remember the potency of each herb. It's not just about flavor, but also about the synergies and interactions of their active compounds.

For instance, blending fennel with other diuretic herbs might amplify the effect, leading to potential dehydration. Thus, understanding each herb's properties is essential in the art of tea blending.

Fennel's Timeless Legacy

As we draw this chapter to a close, the Byzantine world, with its mosaics, hymns, and intricate rituals, might seem distant, but the legacy of fennel, its golden thread in the tapestry of time, connects us to that epoch. Every sip of fennel tea is not just a nod to its health benefits but also a silent toast to the Byzantines, who recognized and venerated its value.

In our cups, the past melds with the present, the boundaries blur, and for a fleeting moment, as the warm liquid touches our lips, we are transported to the echoing halls of Byzantium, where fennel was more than just a herb; it was a symbol, a remedy, a delicacy – a legacy.

Tilia - The Silent Song of Linden

Gentle breezes through the grove,
Tilia's scent, in the air it wove.
Floral notes with a hint of hay,
Whisper of woods where fairies play.

Tilia: A Glimpse into the Verdant World

Majestic and embracing, the linden tree stands tall, its branches extended like the arms of a guardian protector, its leaves whispering tales as ancient as time. Yet it is not just the sight of this tree, but the aroma, the very essence that has captivated humanity for eons.

The Physicality of Tilia

Tilia, commonly known as linden or lime tree (not to be confused with the citrus lime), belongs to the Tiliaceae family. Found predominantly in the temperate regions of the Northern Hemisphere, the linden tree graces the landscapes with its heart-shaped leaves and fragrant yellow-white blossoms. The tree, in its prime, stands as a testament to time, with some living past a millennium. Its bark, textured and telling, and its leaves, serrated at the margins, come together in an architectural marvel of nature.

Origins and Migration: A Journey in Time

The earliest fossils of Tilia date back to the Tertiary period, suggesting an ancient lineage. While its original habitat is believed to be Asia, the linden tree soon spread to Europe and North America. The spread, while a testament to the tree's adaptability, is also an ode to ancient civilizations that recognized its value, carrying its seeds and saplings along with them on their migratory routes.

The Echo of Names: Etymological Tales
Roots in Language

The name 'Tilia' has roots in ancient tongues. Derived from the ancient Greek word 'ptilón', meaning wing, it beautifully captures the essence of the linden tree's winged bract – a modified or specialized leaf – that accompanies its flowers. The term 'linden' is rooted in the Old English 'linde', and the Germanic 'lind', both referring to the flexible nature of the tree, hinting at its use in crafting and carving.

Yet, names, like history, evolve, and with each civilization, the linden tree took on a new moniker, each reflecting its relationship with the people and its significance in their culture.

A Symphony of Senses: Aroma and Taste
The Fragrant Dance

The true allure of Tilia doesn't lie just in its visual splendor, but in its olfactory embrace. As summer arrives, the blossoms unfurl, releasing an intoxicating, sweet scent. This aroma, delicate yet persistent, wafts through the summer air, drawing bees and humans alike.

This scent, when translated into the tea, morphs into a floral, honey-like fragrance, often accompanied by a hint of green, fresh hay. It's an aroma that doesn't scream but whispers, inviting one to lean in, to listen, to engage.

On the Palate

Linden tea offers a gentle embrace. On the palate, its taste mirrors its aroma – notes of honey and floral sweetness, underpinned by a subtle woody undertone. The mouthfeel is smooth, almost silky, making each sip a luxurious experience.

Unlike robust black teas or the grassiness of green teas, linden tea is subtle, a soft serenade compared to a boisterous ballad. It's a tea that demands mindfulness, urging the drinker to be in the moment, to savor and experience rather than just drink.

The Heartland of Europe: Lithuania's Resonant Past

Breath of the Baltic

Tucked away in the northeastern contours of Europe, sharing its coast with the icy embrace of the Baltic Sea, Lithuania stands as a guardian of ancient traditions. A nation whose history oscillates between formidable grand duchies and oppressive occupations, Lithuania is as resilient as the age-old linden trees that grace its landscapes.

Lithuania's narrative isn't linear. Its tale is one of ebbs and flows, of rises and falls. But beneath the veneer of historical upheavals, a deeper cultural vein thrummed, pulsating with age-old traditions, rituals, and an unwavering bond with nature.

Brewing Heritage: The Linden's Embrace in Lithuania

More Than Just A Tree

In Lithuania, as in many parts of Europe, the linden tree is not merely flora; it's an emblem of cultural identity. In villages and towns, it's common to find a linden tree standing tall, sometimes at the heart of community gatherings. Such was its importance that many Lithuanian folk songs, or 'dainos', crooned of the linden tree, intertwining its existence with tales of love, heroism, and nature.

Tilia's Role in Rituals and Healing

The sacredness of Tilia in Lithuanian culture is palpable. Traditionally, it was believed that the tree could ward off evil spirits. Often, linden trees were planted around churches, homes, and graveyards. Their presence was considered a shield, a protective aura against malevolent forces.

Moreover, the ancient Lithuanians, deeply attuned to the rhythms of nature, recognized the healing properties of the linden tree. Long before Linden tea became a staple in modern European households, Lithuanian healers, or 'žyniai', brewed the leaves and blossoms of the linden tree, prescribing its gentle elixir for various ailments.

The Communal Brew: Tilia in Lithuanian Festivities

In the balmy embrace of midsummer, as Lithuania gears up to celebrate 'Joninės', or the Midsummer festival, also known locally as Rasos, the linden tree assumes a role of paramount significance. As fires crackle and songs resonate, linden branches, bedecked with blossoms, are woven into crowns. These crowns, worn especially by young women, symbolize purity and are a nod to the age-old reverence for Tilia.

But beyond adornments, the midsummer festival also witnesses the brewing of Linden tea. As dusk gives way to a night that's scarcely dark, owing to Lithuania's geographical location, communal pots simmer with the fragrant brew. The tea, sipped under a sky ablaze with stars, serves not just as a beverage, but as a link to the past, a silent toast to ancestors, and a nod to nature's bounty.

From Folklore to Pharmacology: The Modern-Day Relevance of Linden Tea

While linden tea's cultural significance in Lithuania is evident, its relevance isn't merely historical or ritualistic. Modern pharmacology, in its quest to decode nature's mysteries, has shone a spotlight on the myriad benefits of Linden tea.

Heartfelt Benefits

Linden tea, with its smooth texture and floral notes, is more than just a sensory delight. Several studies have pointed to its potential role in reducing hypertension. The compounds in linden blossoms exhibit vasodilatory effects, aiding in the relaxation of blood vessels, potentially offering solace to a stressed cardiovascular system.

In an era where the mind often races faster than the clock, the calming effects of linden tea come as a balm. Traditionally, Lithuanian elders often recommended a cup of linden tea to soothe frayed nerves. Today, this age-old wisdom finds an echo in modern research, with studies suggesting that the flavonoids in linden tea may have mild anxiolytic effects.

The Side Effects

While linden tea is generally considered safe, it's essential to recognize that like all herbal remedies, it's not without its caveats. In excessive amounts, linden tea might lead to heart problems, given its profound effect on the cardiovascular system. Additionally, those with known allergies might exhibit hypersensitivity to linden blossoms.

Alchemy in a Teacup: Interactions with Other Herbal Brews

Blending teas isn't merely an art; it's also science. When linden tea mingles with other herbal brews, the symphony can be harmonious or cacophonous, depending on the blend.

For instance, when paired with chamomile, another calming herb, the blend can enhance the soothing effects, making it an ideal nighttime brew. However, blending linden with stimulant herbs, like ginseng, might counteract its calming properties.

In the tapestry of Lithuania's history, the linden tree weaves a thread of cultural heritage, offering a cup of serenity, a sip of tradition, and a taste of nature's enduring wisdom. The journey of Tilia's tea, from ancient rituals to modern mugs, stands as a testament to the enduring bond between a nation and its herbal heritage.

Holy Basil – The Sacred Stress Reliever

From aroma to taste, a journey profound,
In Tulsi's embrace, tranquility is found.
A gift from the heavens, to earth it came,
A sip of the sacred, life's gentle flame.

Unveiling Tulsi: Nature's Verdant Queen

Genesis of a Green Goddess

Holy Basil, with its small, delicate leaves and potent fragrance, isn't just any plant in the vast botanical universe. In the vastness of India—a country as diverse in its ecology as in its cultures—Tulsi stands apart. This isn't merely a plant; it's a symbol, an emblem of both the divine and the therapeutic.

Its roots, both literal and metaphorical, delve deep into the subcontinent's soil, drawing nourishment from millennia of cultural, spiritual, and medicinal traditions.

Etymological Echoes: Naming the Divine

The word 'Tulsi' is derived from Sanskrit, a language as ancient as the civilization itself. It translates to "the incomparable one", a name fitting for a plant revered not just for its therapeutic properties but also for its sacral significance in Hindu mythology.

Notes of Nectar: Tulsi's Aroma and Taste Profile

Fragrance from the Heavens

To understand Tulsi's aroma is to embark on a sensory journey across India. Close your eyes, and you're transported to the heart of monsoon-drenched courtyards in traditional homes, where a Tulsi plant reigns supreme, its fragrance mingling with the petrichor. It's a scent that's at once earthy and divine, grounding and uplifting.

Tulsi's aroma is a complex tapestry. It carries the sharpness of peppermint, the depth of clove, and hints of licorice. It's a scent that lingers, a fragrant reminder of the plant's potent presence.

Elixirs of Echoing Eons

A sip of Tulsi tea is a communion with antiquity. It's sharp, with a peppery kick that gives way to subtle sweetness, an aftertaste that soothes and lingers. But drinking Tulsi tea isn't just a sensory experience; it's a ritual, a moment of pause, a nod to traditions that have, for centuries, celebrated this verdant brew.

Historical Leaves: The Journey of Holy Basil

From Vedic Verses to Modern Mornings

The Vedic texts, ancient scriptures written in the early days of Indian civilization, are replete with references to Tulsi. These texts, which form the bedrock of much of India's spiritual, cultural, and medicinal ethos, celebrated Tulsi not just as a divine entity but also as a healer, a protector against maladies.

Historically, the journey of Tulsi is intertwined with India's own evolution. As kingdoms rose and fell, as dynasties came and went, Tulsi remained a constant. Emperors and paupers, priests and laymen, all turned to this humble plant for solace, be it spiritual or physical.

Trade, Tales, and Tulsi

While Tulsi's heartland was undeniably the Indian subcontinent, its tale doesn't remain confined there. As Indian traders ventured out, they took with them spices, textiles, and tales of Tulsi. It found takers in ancient Greece, where it was known as the "King of Herbs." In Chinese traditional medicine, too, Tulsi made its presence felt, lauded for its unique properties.

The Silk Road, that ancient highway of commerce and culture, played a pivotal role in Tulsi's journey. Caravans laden with goods would often carry dried Tulsi leaves, introducing this Indian marvel to distant lands.

The Canvas of Indian Civilization

The Indian subcontinent, vast and varied, is a cauldron of cultures, religions, and epochs. Here, the mighty Himalayas stand guard in the north, while the southern tips are caressed by three seas. Civilizations flourished on the fertile plains of the Indus and the Ganges, leaving behind legacies that would shape the course of world history.

The Indus Valley and the Vedas

One cannot begin an odyssey into Indian civilization without acknowledging the advanced urban realms of the Indus Valley. It was in the cradle of this ancient civilization, around 3300 BCE, that intricate city planning, undeciphered scripts, and terracotta sculptures emerged. It is also believed that early concepts of health, well-being, and herbal remedies were sown here.

Then came the Vedic age, with sacred hymns echoing through forests and across rivers. Comprising the oldest scriptures of Hinduism, the Vedas laid down rituals, philosophies, and the basis for Ayurveda – India's ancient system of medicine.

Sacred Sips: Tulsi in the Indian Epoch

Divine Origins

India's engagement with Holy Basil, or Tulsi, is deeply spiritual. Rooted in Hindu mythology, the plant is venerated as an earthly manifestation of the goddess Tulsi, a devoted wife to Lord Vishnu and an embodiment of piety. Folk tales and scriptures brim with her tales, weaving Tulsi into the fabric of Indian spirituality.

The Ceremonial Chalice: Drinking to Divinity

Tulsi tea, while therapeutic, also held ceremonial importance. During religious rituals, leaves of the Tulsi plant would be offered to deities, particularly Vishnu, symbolizing surrender, devotion, and the purification of the soul. In many traditional homes, a 'Tulsi Vrindavan' – a special masonry structure – stands in courtyards, where daily offerings, including water infused with Tulsi leaves, are made.

The act of consuming Tulsi tea, for many, goes beyond mere ingestion; it is a sacral communion, imbibing blessings and imbibing health.

A Therapeutic Treasure: Tulsi's Medicinal Might

Ayurveda and the Holy Basil

Ayurveda, translated as the 'science of life,' predates modern medicine by centuries. This ancient Indian system places emphasis on the balance of bodily energies (doshas) and employs natural remedies, including herbs like Tulsi, to maintain equilibrium.

Tulsi's therapeutic prowess in Ayurveda is unparalleled. Labelled as an 'adaptogen,' the plant aids in combating stress and balancing the body's metabolic processes. Its leaves, when consumed as tea, are believed to fortify the immune system, support respiratory health, and counteract environmental toxins.

Modern Science Meets Ancient Wisdom

In contemporary times, research has endeavored to understand Tulsi through the lens of modern medicine. Studies indicate that compounds in Tulsi leaves, such as eugenol, camphene, and cineole, possess anti-inflammatory and antioxidant properties. When sipped as a tea, Tulsi might act as a tonic for the nervous system and a moderator of blood glucose levels.

A Concoction's Caution

While Tulsi tea holds a revered position in India's cultural and medicinal tapestry, it's essential to tread with awareness. Like all potent herbs, Tulsi too has its caveats.

Pregnant or nursing women, for instance, are often advised to limit their consumption of Tulsi tea. The herb, with its powerful compounds, might influence hormone levels, affecting reproductive health. Those on medications for diabetes or hypertension should exercise caution, as Tulsi may amplify the effects of these drugs.

Blends and Bonds: Interactions with Other Herbs

In the vast world of herbal teas, combinations and concoctions abound. Tulsi, with its distinctive taste and therapeutic profile, can be blended with various herbs to enhance both flavor and function.

Mingle with Mint: The sharpness of mint coupled with the warmth of Tulsi creates a refreshing blend, often aiding digestion. *Camomile Companionship*: When Tulsi meets camomile, the result is a soothing brew, perfect for relaxation and combating insomnia. *Ginger's Zest*: Combining the spiciness of ginger with Tulsi's depth offers an immunity-boosting potion, a guard against colds and coughs.

Yet, while blending, one must be aware of the cumulative effects of the herbs. When combining Tulsi with herbs that influence blood sugar, for instance, one must monitor the potential hypoglycemic effects.

In the Quietude of Conclusion

Tulsi – the Holy Basil – isn't just a plant in India; it's an emblem of faith, a testament to the age-old traditions that venerate nature and its myriad gifts. As one sips on a cup of warm, aromatic Tulsi tea, they aren't merely consuming a beverage; they are partaking in a ritual, a legacy, a story that has been brewing for millennia.

The journey of Tulsi, from the sacred scriptures to the modern teacup, is a reflection of India itself – ancient, enduring, and eternally enchanting. And as the last drop is sipped, one can't help but feel a deep sense of gratitude, to nature, to tradition, and to the countless hands that have passed down this green elixir through the corridors of time.

Mugwort - Of Myths and Mists

Bitter at first, then sweetly it lingers,
Mugwort's taste dances on dreamer's fingers.
A sip of the mystical, a touch of the night,
Inviting visions, pure and bright.

The Mugwort: A Botanical Glimpse

Green Shadows of History

The Mugwort, scientifically christened *Artemisia vulgaris*, holds an ancient and enigmatic position in the annals of plant lore. A perennial, with dark green, pinnate leaves and red-purple stems, the plant grows across temperate zones of Europe, Asia, and Northern Africa. It proudly unfurls its leaves, often in places left wild and untouched – along roadsides, riverbanks, and hedgerows.

Etymological Echoes

The name 'Mugwort' conjures images that are simultaneously rustic and mystical. Delving into its etymology, the term 'mug' is believed to stem from the Old Norse 'muggi', signifying a marsh or a fen, possibly referencing the plant's predilection for damp soils. The 'wort' is a vestige of Old English, an affix given to plants with utilitarian value, akin to root or herb.

From Bud to Brew: A Sensory Experience

Aroma: A Gateway to Another Era

Mugwort, when crushed between fingers, releases an aroma that is a blend of the earthy and the ethereal. There's a hint of sage, a whiff of camphor, and a lingering trace of woods after rainfall. This aroma is a transportive agent, capable of whisking one away to an ancient forest, where druids once tread and where spirits might still dwell.

Flavor: The Arcane in a Sip

Mugwort tea, when brewed, invites with its warm amber hue. The first sip might be a jolt – an unexpected bitter note, not entirely unwelcome but certainly commanding attention. As the palate adjusts, underlying complexities emerge: a subtle sweetness, akin to dried fruit or a dark honey, followed by an earthy undertone reminiscent of wet leaves or moss.

The Precarious Dance of Bitter and Sweet

The beauty of Mugwort tea lies in its duality. This is not a tea for passive consumption; it is a tea that demands engagement. As the bitterness and sweetness dance on the tongue, they tell a tale of nature's balances and of ancient rituals where Mugwort was central.

Bitterness, often shunned in modern culinary endeavors, was once prized – seen as a sign of potency and medicinal might. And in the bitterness of Mugwort, there's a callback to times when herbs were revered not just for their flavor, but for their inherent power to heal, protect, or divine.

From its undulating growth beside untouched pathways to the rich tapestry of its sensory experience, Mugwort is a plant steeped in mystique. It is a bridge, connecting us to the old ways, to whispered legends, and to nature's enigmatic heart.

As the last traces of its aroma fade, and the final sip leaves the cup, one thing becomes evident: Mugwort tea is not just a beverage; it is an experience, a rite, and a journey into the arcane alcoves of history and the soul.

The Floating World of Japan

In the heart of the Far East lies an island nation of profound contrasts: Japan. From snow-capped Mount Fuji to verdant bamboo forests, its land is a canvas of nature's artistry. But to understand Mugwort's place within this tapestry, one must first delve into the psyche of a civilization that, for centuries, has effortlessly blended the ancient with the avant-garde.

Whispers of the Shinto Spirits

The Kami and Nature's Embrace

To begin to fathom the significance of Mugwort within Japanese culture, we turn first to Shintoism – the indigenous faith of the Japanese. Shinto, or 'the way of the gods', doesn't just revere deities. It celebrates *kami*, spirits found in objects and phenomena. The rustling of leaves, the bubbling of springs, the towering presence of ancient trees – all are evidence of *kami* at play.

Within this framework, plants aren't merely botanical entities; they are living, breathing embodiments of the divine. This perspective offers a lens through which the Japanese appreciation for Mugwort – known as *yomogi* in local parlance – can be more deeply understood.

The Brewed Chronicles of *Yomogi*

The Ritual of Kuchikami

In the annals of ancient Japan, there are references to a unique form of sake brewing, known as *kuchikami*, or 'mouth-chewed'. This method involved village maidens chewing rice, chestnuts, or millet and spitting the mixture into tubs. Natural enzymes in the saliva facilitated fermentation. Into this mix, various herbs, including Mugwort, were introduced, not only for flavor but for spiritual potency.

Yomogi in such concoctions was believed to protect drinkers from malevolent spirits, perhaps a nod to the plant's widespread reputation across cultures as a protective herb.

Mochi and the Springtime Blessings

No discussion of Mugwort in Japan can be complete without acknowledging *yomogi mochi*. This delicacy, consumed during spring, comprises a chewy rice cake filled with sweet red bean paste, with the dough infused with the green essence of Mugwort. It's not just a treat; it's a ritual – a celebration of the changing seasons and the rejuvenation that spring promises.

Modern Elixirs and Ancient Echoes

Beyond Folklore: The Therapeutic Tapestry

Though the tales of spirits and protective rites might be relegated to folklore, the benefits of Mugwort are palpably present. Modern science, with its tools and metrics, finds in this herb compounds that echo the wisdom of ancients.

Consuming Mugwort tea is linked to digestive health. Its bitter compounds stimulate the production of bile, aiding digestion. Additionally, the herb's nervine properties make it an ally for those grappling with anxiety or insomnia.

Side Effects and Interactions

Yet, every elixir has its limits. And while Mugwort is a treasure trove of benefits, it's not without its caveats. Prolonged consumption can lead to side effects, such as allergies or, in rare instances, hallucinogenic dreams. Pregnant women are advised to steer clear, as compounds in Mugwort can stimulate the uterus.

When Mugwort meets other herbs in a blend, the dance is intricate. With chamomile, it might enhance sleep-inducing effects. With peppermint, it can further bolster digestive benefits. But with valerian or hops, the sedative effects could be exaggerated, warranting caution.

In the Brewed Depths of Reflection

If history were a tapestry, Japan's thread would shimmer uniquely, iridescent with tales of emperors and samurais, of cherry blossoms and silent Zen gardens. Within this weave, *yomogi* finds its delicate trace, linking the realm of spirits with that of the mortal, the ancient with the present.

In the end, Mugwort tea is more than a brew. In Japan, it's a sip of history, a draught of culture, and a whisper of spirits long revered but never forgotten. The dance of *yomogi* through Japan's chronicles is a testament to a culture's ability to honor tradition while embracing transformation.

Valerian – The Whispering Root

From earth's embrace to the moon's soft glow,
Valerian's taste lets the mind slow.
A gentle bitterness, a tranquil treat,
A flavor that makes the night complete.

The Enigma of the Valerian Root

In the verdant embrace of Europe and Asia, a perennial plant unfurls its feathery leaves, waiting for the touch of summer to bloom with pale-pink blossoms. Known as Valeriana officinalis to the botanist and valerian to the common folk, this plant's humble appearance belies its potent legacy.

From Rome to Medieval Europe: A Plant's Journey Through Time

Valeriana: The Etymological Conundrum

Etymology often presents us with fascinating windows into a word's past, and valerian is no exception. Some posit that its name is derived from the Latin word "valere," meaning "to be healthy" or "to be strong," apt for a herb long associated with therapeutic properties. Others speculate a connection to the Roman Emperor Valerian (Publius Licinius Valerianus), but historical records linking the emperor directly to the herb remain elusive.

A Scent Unlike Any Other

One cannot engage with valerian without noting its distinctive aroma. To say it's an acquired taste is an understatement. While the flowers might seduce bees with their sweet scent, the roots tell a different olfactory story – musky, woody, and, to some, reminiscent of worn socks. Yet, this off-putting scent is where much of valerian's magic resides.

The Embodied Taste of Tradition

To sip valerian tea is to partake in a ritual older than many civilizations. The taste, earthy and slightly bitter, is often softened with other herbs in modern preparations, but to experience it in its undiluted form is to understand its ancient appeal – a deep, grounding connection to the earth from which it springs.

Arabia and the Spice Routes: Valerian's Eastern Odyssey

As with many botanical tales, valerian's journey is intertwined with the desires and destinies of human civilizations. And to chart its course, one must voyage to the aromatic world of the Arabian Peninsula.

The Desert's Liquid Gold

While Arabia's fragrant contribution to the world is often distilled in the essence of frankincense and myrrh, its aromatic tapestry is far richer. Valerian, though not native to the region, found its way into the pharmacopeia of medieval Arab physicians.

Alchemy and Healing: Arabic Innovations

Arab scholars, inheriting the vast compendiums of Greek and Roman knowledge, weren't just content preserving ancient wisdom. They expanded upon it. The great Persian polymath Avicenna, in his monumental work *Canon of Medicine*, mentions valerian's utility, particularly emphasizing its benefits for the nervous system.

It's no coincidence that as Europe languished in the Dark Ages, the Islamic world experienced a renaissance, with valerian playing a small yet significant role in the grander tapestry of its medical advancements.

From Root to Cup: Modern Concoctions and Age-old Remedies

Valerian's journey from a wild-growing herb to a staple in modern wellness wasn't straightforward. Its adoption, particularly in the West, owes much to the Arabic world's meticulous documentation and experimentation.

Valerian Today: Health in a Teacup

Modern science, with its penchant for validation, has found several of valerian's traditional uses to be efficacious. Chief among these is its role in promoting sleep and reducing anxiety. The compounds in valerian, especially valerenic acid, have been shown to increase the release of a neurotransmitter called gamma-aminobutyric acid (GABA), which has a calming effect on anxiety and helps regulate the sleep cycle.

A Brew with Caveats

As with many potent remedies, valerian requires respect in its consumption. While generally safe for most, some people might experience dizziness, upset stomach, or dry mouth. It's also worth noting that chronic use can lead to withdrawal symptoms, underscoring the importance of moderation.

Interactions and Synergies: Crafting the Perfect Blend

Valerian's powerful calming properties can be both a blessing and a challenge when combined with other herbs. In blends with chamomile or lemon balm, its sleep-inducing effects can be amplified. However, combined with herbs like St. John's Wort, there's a risk of excessive sedation.

Arabia: A Tapestry of Time and Tradition

In the vast stretches of the Arabian deserts, where the sand seems to merge with the sky, emerged a civilization rooted in the wisdom of sages and the tales of traders. Here, where ancient caravan routes crisscrossed like veins, knowledge was the true wealth, sought with the same fervor as gold or frankincense. And among this treasure trove of information was the humble valerian.

Alchemy of Arabia: The Dawn of a Medical Renaissance

The Islamic Golden Age and Medicine

It is essential to appreciate the broader context in which valerian thrived in the Arabic world. The period, often referred to as the Islamic Golden Age, spanning the 8th to the 13th century, saw a blossoming of science, philosophy, and medicine. And at this crossroad of civilizations - where Greek, Indian, Persian, and Egyptian thought converged - the Arabic scholars played a pivotal role in synthesizing and advancing global knowledge.

Valerian: The Silent Soother

Though valerian's journey began in Europe and Asia, it was in the bustling bazaars and hallowed halls of Arabic academia that it found an elevated status.

The Manuscripts and Monographs

Several ancient Arabic medical treatises extol the virtues of valerian. While earlier references may have been primarily centered on its aromatic properties, soon its sedative qualities were recognized and documented.

Notably, the renowned Persian polymath, Avicenna, in his seminal work, *The Canon of Medicine*, elucidated valerian's therapeutic properties. To Avicenna and his peers, the root was more than just a soporific aid; it was a panacea for the nervous system, addressing ailments from insomnia to seizures.

Soulful Infusions: The Spiritual Essence of Valerian

While the West often demarcates the spiritual from the medicinal, the Arabic world, especially in its golden age, saw them as intertwined. In this milieu, valerian was not just a root, but a conduit to inner tranquility.

Echoes in the Qur'an?

While the Qur'an doesn't directly mention valerian, its emphasis on plants as divine signs is evident. Given the prominence of valerian in medical and possibly spiritual circles, it might have been implicitly celebrated as one of the many botanical wonders gifted by the divine.

Dreams, Divinity, and Valerian

Arabian nights are as famed for their celestial beauty as they are for tales told under their starry embrace. Dreams held a special place in Arabic culture, often seen as omens or divine messages. With valerian's properties inducing vivid dreams, its consumption might have been ritualized, not merely for its calming effects but as an aid to spiritual communion.

Valerian in the Modern Arabic Repertoire

While the bustling scientific fervor of the Golden Age may have dimmed, the traditions and knowledge of that era still echo in the modern Arabic world, particularly in the realm of herbal remedies.

Contemporary Concoctions

Today, valerian is frequently found in households across the Middle East, not just as a remedy for sleep disturbances, but also as a go-to solution for anxiety and stress. Modern medicine, with its array of drugs, hasn't dimmed valerian's allure in the region. Its natural roots (quite literally) make it a preferred choice for many who seek solutions grounded in tradition.

The Many Faces of Valerian: Boons and Banes

As with many gifts of nature, valerian's embrace comes with its caveats. While the root offers solace to many, it demands respect in its consumption.

Side Effects and Sensitivities

Though largely benign, valerian isn't without its quirks. Overconsumption can lead to an array of symptoms, from the mild (headaches, digestive disturbances) to the more concerning (liver damage in rare cases). Additionally, its prolonged use can lead to withdrawal symptoms, akin to those experienced with sedative medications.

Synergies and Interactions

Valerian's sedative prowess can be both a gift and a challenge, especially when blended with other herbs. When paired with the likes of chamomile or lemon balm, the result can be a deeply calming brew. However, caution is advised when combining it with other potent herbs or medications, as the effects can be cumulative.

The Arabian Legacy

The story of valerian in Arabia isn't just the tale of a herb. It's a narrative of a civilization's pursuit of knowledge and well-being, a journey from the starlit deserts to the scholarly halls of Baghdad and Cordoba. Valerian, with its silent soothing powers, stands as a testament to the Arabic world's timeless commitment to healing, both of the body and the soul. And as the night descends upon the Arabian sands, under the watchful eyes of the stars, one can almost hear the whispers of the ancients, singing praises of this wondrous root.

Cinnamon's Allure - From Forests to Fragrant Brews

A dance of fire upon the tongue,
Cinnamon's warmth has tales unsung.
A fusion of sweet and fiery zest,
Each sip feels like a festive jest.

The Bark that Brews: The Cinnamomum Verum

Introducing the Cinnamomum

Behind the golden-brown swirls of cinnamon lies the tree *Cinnamomum verum*, an evergreen native to the heart of Sri Lanka. Though it has several siblings in the *Cinnamomum* family, it is this particular tree that gives us the most prized of cinnamon. Cloaked in a rough exterior, its inner bark, when peeled away and dried, curls into the familiar quills that have perfumed kitchens and sanctums for millennia.

Tracing Origins: Beyond the Bounds of Time

Unearthing the Etymology

Cinnamon, or as the ancient Greeks called it, 'kinnámōmon', is more than just a word; it's a historical tapestry woven with threads from various cultures. Tracing its linguistic roots, one discovers layers of its journey - from the ancient Phoenician traders who introduced it to the Greeks, to the Hebrew Bible, where it was mentioned as 'qinnamon', hinting at its coveted status even in those ancient times.

The Historical Harvest

To chart the history of cinnamon is to traverse through a dense forest, with trails both known and speculative. Ancient Egyptians utilized it in their mummification rituals, and it found its way into early Chinese writings as far back as 2800 BCE. But while its presence in these ancient civilizations is documented, the exact origins remain shrouded in mystery. Early on, cinnamon was so highly esteemed that it was considered a fitting gift for monarchs and even divinities.

Sensory Symphony: The Aroma and the Ambrosia

The Enchanting Aroma

One can't speak of cinnamon without indulging in its aromatic allure. Warm, sweet, and slightly woody, the fragrance of cinnamon is unmistakably captivating. The science behind its scent lies in its essential oil, notably cinnamaldehyde, which accounts for over 60% of its essential oil composition. When released, either through grinding or brewing, it's this compound that we have to thank for the olfactory embrace that fills the air.

The Tantalizing Taste

To the tongue, cinnamon is a tapestry of tastes – its inherent sweetness, interlaced with a hint of spice, evokes both comfort and intrigue. It's a warmth that spreads, not just in the mouth, but through the very soul, making it a cherished addition to both savory and sweet dishes. However, when transformed into tea, cinnamon offers a delicate balance – a gentle sweetness paired with an almost citrusy brightness.

The Cradle of Civilization: Mesopotamia Briefed

In the interlaced rivers of the Tigris and Euphrates, history was being written long before the art of writing even came into being. Mesopotamia, often heralded as the 'cradle of civilization,' was the seat of empires, the harbinger of writing systems, and a melting pot of cultures. Spanning modern-day Iraq, parts of Iran, Syria, and Turkey, this region was the birthplace of cities and civilization as we know it.

Settlements to Empires

From the Sumerians to the Assyrians, the Akkadians to the Babylonians, Mesopotamia's civilization tapestry was richly woven with intricacies. City-states like Ur, Uruk, and Eridu, which started as humble settlements, grew in power and influence, controlling vast tracts of land, navigating intricate trade routes, and waging wars.

The Mesopotamian Palate: More than Bread and Beer

The land between two rivers was fertile, allowing agriculture to flourish. While Mesopotamians are often associated with their staples like barley-made bread and beer, their diet was elaborate and diverse. Culinary sophistication was apparent in their use of herbs, spices, and flavorings, making their dishes both flavorful and therapeutic.

Cinnamon's Sojourn to Mesopotamia

Trade and the Cinnamon Route

Long before the famed Silk Road, there was the cinnamon route. Originating in the rainforests of Sri Lanka, cinnamon had to pass through countless hands, traverse vast lands, and cross treacherous seas before reaching the Mesopotamian shores. Given its distance from the source, cinnamon was not just another spice for Mesopotamians—it was an exotic luxury.

The Mesopotamian Infusion: Brewing Traditions

Although it's hard to pinpoint when exactly cinnamon made its debut in Mesopotamian tea pots, records and cuneiform tablets suggest its valued presence. Did the Sumerians savor a primitive form of cinnamon tea? It's possible. Evidence suggests that they boiled various herbs and spices to make infusions, not very different from today's teas.

Spiritual or Secular: The Significance of Cinnamon

Gifts for the Gods

Cinnamon's exotic nature and fragrant profile meant it was more than just a culinary delight—it had spiritual significance. In the Mesopotamian pantheon, offerings to the gods were an integral part of religious practices. It wasn't uncommon for precious spices like cinnamon to be offered at the altars of gods such as Marduk and Inanna.

On the secular front, cinnamon found its way into the homes of the elite. The middle and upper echelons of Mesopotamian society, with their access to imported goods, would have been the primary consumers of this luxurious spice. Infused in their teas or sprinkled on their dishes, cinnamon was a symbol of status.

The Timeless Brew: Health Benefits and Modern Understandings

From Ancient Remedies to Modern Science

Mesopotamian physicians, hailed as *asu*, often combined the roles of both priest and doctor. They believed in the balance of spirits and used a mix of prayers and medicinal herbs to treat ailments. Cinnamon, with its aromatic compounds, was likely prized for its perceived health benefits. Fast forward to today, and modern science affirms some of these ancient beliefs. Cinnamon has been found to have anti-inflammatory properties, can aid in blood sugar control, and boasts antioxidants.

Potential Side Effects

No matter the elixir, moderation is key. While cinnamon tea is largely benign, overconsumption, especially of the Cassia variant, can lead to a buildup of coumarin, a natural compound which, in large doses, may cause liver damage. Furthermore, excessive cinnamon can lead to mouth sores or an allergic reaction in some sensitive individuals.

A Symphony of Flavors: Cinnamon and Its Herbal Comrades

In the world of herbal teas, blends are the magic that results when different herbs dance together in a cup. Cinnamon, with its warm and sweet profile, is often blended with other herbs. Paired with ginger, it amplifies warmth; with chamomile, it adds a layer of depth. However, it's essential to understand individual herbs before blending, ensuring that their benefits align and do not counteract one another.

Conclusion: Cinnamon - Mesopotamia's Liquid Gold

In the annals of Mesopotamian history, amidst tales of kings, gods, and wars, cinnamon quietly brewed its own legacy. From the bustling markets of Babylon to the sacred altars of Sumer, it was more than just a spice—it was a fragment of the exotic, a whiff of the divine. And as we sip our cinnamon tea today, we are, in essence, savoring a brew that once graced the tables of ancient Mesopotamia, a testament to the timeless allure of cinnamon.

Mate – The Elixir of Vigor

The South's gift to the waking morn,
Mate revives like a new day born.
Its zestful taste, both sharp and true,
Ignites passion and vigor anew.

The Sacred Leaf: Yerba Mate

From the dense, emerald-hued forests of South America rises a legacy – not just of a plant, but of an entire culture. The *Ilex paraguariensis*, a tall, resilient tree, stands amidst the other flora, but it's the tree's leaves and stems that have carved a niche in history and our cups. These leaves, when dried and processed, become the main ingredient of the invigorating drink we call mate.

One can easily overlook the cultural tapestry intertwined with mate's history. At the outset, it is just another tea. But as you delve deeper, you understand the sanctity this beverage has held for countless generations, becoming an indelible part of South America's socio-cultural narrative.

Etymological Roots: A Glimpse into Origins

The term "mate" finds its origin in the Quechua word "matí", which translates to "cup". This is no mere coincidence. The traditional method of consuming this tea requires a hollowed-out calabash gourd, signifying the vessel that contains the essence of nature.

Yet, it's not just the name of the drink but also the ritualistic consumption that evokes a sense of community.

The very act of sharing a mate drink, passing it around, makes it more than a mere beverage; it's a symbol of unity, friendship, and tradition.

A Symphony of Aroma and Taste

The experience of drinking mate is a sensory journey. The initial aroma is a potent mix of earthy woods with a hint of tobacco. Depending on the processing, some might even sense a mild smokiness. This isn't the vegetative scent that you associate with green teas; it's deeper, wilder, like the very forests from which it originates.

Upon the first sip, a new world unfolds. Mate's taste, robust and unparalleled, is a blend of its forested origin. There's the primary bitter note, reminiscent of well-steeped dark teas. But then come the undertones. The subtle sweetness, the grassy freshness, the hints of spice, and a soft, lingering tartness.

Yet, what makes mate stand apart is its after-effect. Unlike other teas, mate doesn't just refresh; it invigorates. There's a burst of energy, an awakening of the senses – as if the very spirit of the forests is coursing through you.

Beyond the Cup: The Processing of Mate

To understand mate's unique aroma and flavor profile, it's essential to dive into its preparation. After harvesting, the leaves are often blanched or steamed to halt the enzymatic process. They're then dried – traditionally by a wood fire, which imparts that unique smoky undertone.

Post drying, the leaves might be aged, sometimes for years. Aging allows the flavors to mature, to deepen. It mellows down the initial bitterness and brings out the nuanced sweetness. However, not all mate is aged; fresh mate, called "Yerba Mate Verde," is green and retains a stronger grassy note.

The World of the Guaraní

To venture into the world of the Guaraní is to walk amidst the luscious green corridors of South America's forests. Spread across what we now call Paraguay, Brazil, Argentina, and Bolivia, the Guaraní were among the first people to cultivate and consume the drink that Mate has come to be.

As we sink into the deeper layers of history, a vivacious picture of the Guaraní emerges. Here was a semi-nomadic tribe, their existence seamlessly interwoven with nature. The forests were not just their home but an extension of their very being. The symbiotic relationship they shared with nature defined their culture, spirituality, and daily routines.

Mate: Beyond a Beverage

Within the Guaraní culture, Mate was never just a drink. Instead, it represented a complex tapestry of spiritual beliefs, societal rituals, and an acknowledgment of nature's profound gifts.

The Spiritual Brew: For the Guaraní, everything had a spirit – the trees, the animals, the rivers, and the winds. These spirits were not mere figments of folklore; they were palpable entities, interlacing daily life. Mate, derived from the sacred tree, was thus seen as a direct link to the divine world. The act of drinking Mate was a communion, a conversation between the mortal and the spirits.

Ritualistic Bonds: While the spiritual aspects of Mate were paramount, its societal implications cannot be understated. Sharing a gourd of Mate was a ritual, an affirmation of trust and camaraderie. Leaders would discuss pressing matters over a shared gourd, families would bond over it, and disputes would be settled. To share a Mate was to share one's life.

The Medicinal Elixir

The Guaraní's understanding of Mate wasn't restricted to its spiritual facets. Their intimate knowledge of the forest translated to an intrinsic understanding of Mate's health benefits.

Natural Energizer: The Guaraní warriors often consumed Mate before heading into battles or embarking on long journeys. They believed it endowed them with heightened stamina, allowing them to travel days without feeling the weight of fatigue.

Digestive Aid: While they didn't possess the scientific jargon of our times, the Guaraní recognized Mate's role in aiding digestion. After communal feasts, a gourd of Mate was passed around, ensuring the tribe felt light and agile.

From Ancient Traditions to Modern Realizations

Mate's journey from the sacred forests of the Guaraní to global recognition is a testament to its undeniable qualities.

Health and Beyond: Today, science validates what the Guaraní have known for centuries. Mate is rich in antioxidants, potentially more than even green tea. It's known to boost metabolism, aid digestion, and enhance physical endurance. Its unique combination of caffeine, theobromine, and theophylline makes it a stimulant that rejuvenates without the jitters associated with coffee.

The Cautionary Note: As with anything, moderation is the key. Excessive consumption of Mate, especially when consumed very hot, has been linked to potential health risks. It's also essential to recognize that while Mate invigorates, it should not replace rest or be consumed to push the body beyond its natural limits.

The Blending Ballet

Mate, with its distinct flavor profile, often dances solo in a cup. But, its interaction with other herbal infusions creates a medley of sensory experiences.

Mate and Mint: When the freshness of mint meets the depth of Mate, a cooling yet invigorating blend emerges. This blend is especially popular in certain regions of South America.

Mate and Cocoa: A somewhat modern fusion, yet when the richness of cocoa intertwines with Mate, a beverage reminiscent of a mocha, but with the earthiness of Mate, is born.

Interactions and Caution: While blending Mate can be an exploratory journey, one must be cautious. Combining

Mate with other stimulants might be overwhelming for some. Always be attuned to your body's responses.

As this chapter draws to a close, one recognizes that Mate isn't just a beverage. It is the echo of ancient forests, the whispers of the Guaraní spirits, and the testament of nature's abundant gifts. For the Guaraní, Mate was a bridge – between humans, spirits, and the vast universe. Even today, every sip of Mate is a step on that timeless bridge, reminding us of our roots and the wonders of nature.

Gotu Kola - The Leaf of Longevity

In Whispers of Freshness, In Tones so Mild,
Lies Gotu Kola, Nature's Gift, Forest's Child.
A Sip Transports, To Lush Lands so Green,
Where Time Slows, And Life's Essence is Seen.

The Plant Behind the Potion

In the wetlands and riverbanks across the Asian subcontinent, amidst the cacophony of buzzing insects and distant birdsongs, thrives the Centella asiatica, more fondly known as Gotu Kola. This small perennial herb, with its fan-shaped leaves, may seem ordinary at first glance. But its history and the wealth it brings to our cups are nothing short of extraordinary.

Its roots delve deep into the earth, drawing sustenance from the land's ancient wisdom. Above ground, its green, serrated leaves stretch towards the sky, collecting tales of monsoons and sunrises.

Origins and the Journey of Names

Etymology, often, is the key to a deeper understanding. The term "Gotu Kola" finds its origin in Sinhalese, a language spoken in Sri Lanka. "Gotu" means conical shape, reflecting the herb's leaf structure, and "Kola" translates to leaf. Thus, the very name paints a vivid image of the plant, encapsulating its physical essence.

However, this humble herb has been recognized and revered across various civilizations, each bequeathing it with a name of their own. In traditional Chinese culture, it is known as Ji Xue Cao, which can be translated to 'the herb of memory'.

The Essence: Aroma and Taste

A whiff of Gotu Kola tea often evokes feelings of standing amidst a fresh, dew-kissed meadow at the cusp of dawn. The aroma isn't overpowering but possesses a gentle freshness, a subtle earthiness that hints at its marshy origins.

Upon tasting, one is greeted with a mild, herbaceous flavor. There isn't the boldness that characterizes many teas. Instead, it's a delicate symphony of green notes, with a slight bitterness that is quickly followed by an undertone of sweetness. The overall experience is akin to a gentle embrace by nature, calming and serene.

Gotu Kola in Sri Lankan Lore

Sri Lanka, with its undulating terrains, tropical forests, and golden beaches, is a land steeped in history. Among its ancient temples, traditional dances, and age-old rituals, Gotu Kola occupies a revered place.

In the annals of Sri Lankan traditions, this herb isn't just a plant; it's a repository of legends. Tales of yore often speak of how wise old elephants, known for their longevity, grazed on Gotu Kola, attributing their extended lifespans to this magical herb.

A Culinary and Medicinal Staple

While Gotu Kola tea has grown in popularity in recent times, the herb itself has been an integral part of Sri Lankan cuisine for centuries. The fresh leaves, finely chopped, find their way into savory dishes, salads, and even traditional medicines.

Ayurveda, the ancient Indian system of medicine that also significantly influences Sri Lankan health practices, has long hailed Gotu Kola for its myriad benefits. It was commonly used to treat wounds, improve memory, and even combat anxiety. The local folklore goes that sages with heightened cognitive abilities often consumed Gotu Kola, cementing its reputation as a brain tonic.

The Resonance of an Ancient Civilization

In the sun-kissed islands of the Indian Ocean lies Sri Lanka, a land that bears the weight and wisdom of millennia. With its emerald green landscapes, richly adorned temples, and sonorous folktales, this is a land where every stone and stream narrates a story. Before diving into the herbaceous embrace of Gotu Kola, let us first immerse ourselves in the soul of Sri Lanka.

A Glimpse into Sri Lankan Civilization

The story of Sri Lanka is as layered as the sedimentary rocks that dot its terrains. Inhabited for over 34,000 years, its history is a tapestry woven with threads of Buddhist teachings, Hindu influences, and colonial encounters.

The ancient city of Anuradhapura, now but a collection of ruins and relics, once gleamed as a pinnacle of Sinhalese power. Further south, the rocky fortress of Sigiriya stands as an architectural marvel and a testament to the ingenuity of ancient Sri Lankan civilization.

Yet, amidst the tales of kings and conquests, it's the daily rhythms of life that provide the most evocative stories. In this realm of everyday existence, the Gotu Kola plant emerges as a silent, yet potent protagonist.

Gotu Kola: Beyond the Brew in Sri Lanka

In the labyrinthine alleys of Sri Lankan markets, one can often spot fresh bunches of Gotu Kola leaves, their vibrant green contrasting starkly with the muted browns of the surroundings. To the uninformed observer, these might seem like just another leafy green. But delve deeper, and the narrative unfolds.

For the people of Sri Lanka, Gotu Kola is more than a tea; it's a repository of memories, traditions, and healing. It is a bridge that connects the wisdom of their ancestors to the bustling energy of the present.

Cultural and Spiritual Significance

At the heart of the Sri Lankan ethos lies the profound influence of Buddhism. The teachings of Buddha pervade every aspect of life, from monumental stupas to the simplest of daily routines. In this spiritual milieu, Gotu Kola finds its sanctified space.

Monks, who tread the middle path and seek enlightenment, often incorporate Gotu Kola into their diets. The herb's reputed ability to sharpen the mind and enhance meditation makes it a cherished element in the monastic life. Moreover, folklore is rife with tales of how Gotu Kola aids in achieving the clarity and calmness essential for deep introspection.

Modern Uses and Revelations

Fast forward to the present, and Gotu Kola has transcended its spiritual confines, finding a coveted place in the wellness lexicon. From high-end spas in Colombo to naturopathy centers in the West, the herb is lauded for its myriad benefits.

Brain Booster: One of the most acclaimed benefits of Gotu Kola is its neuroprotective properties. Modern science, with its arsenal of techniques, has reaffirmed what traditional healers professed for centuries: Gotu Kola can potentially aid cognitive function.

Skin Healer: A walk down any Sri Lankan village might reveal local healers using Gotu Kola as a remedy for various skin ailments. Its anti-inflammatory properties make it a popular choice for treating wounds, burns, and even psoriasis.

Adaptogenic Ally: Stress is the malaise of modern existence. Gotu Kola, with its adaptogenic qualities, has emerged as a natural remedy, helping the body adapt to stressors, be they physical, chemical, or biological.

Potential Side Effects

Nature, in its vast bounty, often provides remedies laced with cautions. While Gotu Kola is generally deemed safe, it is not without its nuances. Excessive consumption might lead to headaches, upset stomachs, or even dizziness in some individuals. Pregnant or nursing women, as well as those with liver issues, are advised to approach Gotu Kola with caution.

The Alchemy of Blends

Tea, much like life, is about balance. When Gotu Kola is blended with other herbs, the result is a symphony of flavors and effects. However, this alchemy isn't without its intricacies.

For instance, when combined with herbs like Brahmi (another cognitive enhancer), the effect on mental clarity can be potentiated. However, when mixed with stimulants like green tea or ginseng, it's essential to be cautious, as the combined effect might be too invigorating for some.

In Conclusion: Gotu Kola's Tapestry

Gotu Kola, with its serrated leaves and mild flavor, might seem unassuming. Yet, it stands as a poignant symbol of Sri Lanka's rich heritage, its spiritual pursuits, and its embrace of nature's curatives.

As we navigate the complexities of the modern world, the simple Gotu Kola leaf serves as a reminder of timeless truths. It beckons us to pause, reflect, and find solace in nature's lap, even if it's just for the duration of a tea break. In its gentle embrace, we find both history and hope, tradition and transformation.

Ashwagandha – Adaptogenic Anchor

Bitter meets sweet, a balanced dance,
Each sip a taste of old romance.
Ashwagandha, with its soothing trace,
Brings calm and strength in gentle grace.

Ashwagandha: An Introduction

The world of botanicals brims with mysteries, where each herb and root carries stories older than the most ancient of trees. One such enigma is Ashwagandha, a plant as rooted in history as it is in the fertile soils of the East.

Its scientific name, Withania somnifera, might make it sound like a character from a classical play, but delve a little deeper, and one uncovers tales that span civilizations, epochs, and continents.

Origins and Etymology: The Language of the Earth

To trace the etymology of Ashwagandha is to embark on a linguistic journey through the heart of ancient India. Derived from Sanskrit, 'Ashwa' means 'horse', while 'Gandha' translates to 'smell'. So, the term 'Ashwagandha' can be evocatively interpreted as the 'smell of a horse'. This name speaks volumes about the herb's characteristics, particularly its strong, earthy aroma reminiscent of the vigor and vitality of a stallion.

The root, when freshly dug up, emanates a robust scent. Some say it speaks of the strength it imparts, while others believe it's the very essence of the earth it grows in. Whichever interpretation one leans towards, it's impossible to dissociate Ashwagandha from its potent fragrance.

The Plant: Nature's Resilient Alchemist

Ashwagandha is a shrub. The word 'shrub' might seem too ordinary for a plant with such an illustrious past, but Ashwagandha is a master of humility. With its greenish-yellow flowers, simple leaves, and red berries, it might seem like just another plant. But, like the fabled philosophers' stone, its true magic lies hidden underground.

Its roots, both metaphorically and physically, are where the real story unfolds. These roots, when dried, form the primary ingredient for the legendary Ashwagandha tea.

A Journey of Aromas and Tastes

When it comes to herbal teas, each sip is a tale, and each aroma a chapter. Ashwagandha, in this narrative, offers a compelling plot.

The very first whiff is earthy, almost primal. It's the scent of ancient forests, of lands untouched by modernity. This is closely followed by a subtle sweetness, a fleeting note, almost like a whispered secret.

Upon tasting, the narrative becomes even more layered. The initial flavor profile is a delicate balance of mild bitterness, juxtaposed with hints of natural sweetness. But, like a story with a twist, there's a subtle, warming aftertaste. It lingers, long after the tea has been consumed, much like the memory of a captivating tale.

The Looming Himalayas and the Cradle of Culture

Nepal – a name that evokes images of towering snow-clad peaks, ancient temples, and the undying spirit of its people. Nestled amidst the mighty Himalayas, this nation stands as a testament to the harmony of nature and human endurance.

The grandeur of its geography is matched only by the richness of its culture. A melting pot of ethnicities, religions, and traditions, Nepal's civilization is as intricate as the winding trails that crisscross its landscapes.

Ashwagandha: A Root Deeply Intertwined with Nepalese Heritage

In this landscape, where myths intertwine seamlessly with history, the story of Ashwagandha finds its sacred space.

Sacred Infusions: Ashwagandha and the Spiritual Quest

For the people of Nepal, the realm of the spiritual is as tangible as the looming mountains that surround them. In this world, where deities reside in stones, trees, and rivers, Ashwagandha assumes a divine aura.

While Ashwagandha's primary association is with Ayurveda, its spiritual significance in Nepal is undeniable. Consumed by sages and seers during deep meditative practices, the tea prepared from its roots is believed to instill clarity of mind, deepening one's connection to the ethereal.

Rituals in remote monasteries often included the consumption of Ashwagandha tea to ward off the chilling cold and, more importantly, to keep the mind attuned to the divine frequencies.

Healing the Nepalese Way: Ancient Remedies for Modern Maladies

But beyond the spiritual, Ashwagandha has served as a cornerstone in the everyday lives of the Nepalese. The local healers, known as Vaidyas, often prescribed it as a panacea for a myriad of ailments.

The elderly believed in its power to rejuvenate and restore vitality, while the youth consumed it to enhance physical stamina and mental alertness, crucial in a land where survival often meant battling the elements.

Modern Revelations: Ashwagandha in Contemporary Times

As the world turns its gaze towards organic healing and natural remedies, Ashwagandha has emerged from the shadows of the Himalayan valleys onto the global stage.

Scientific studies now validate what the Nepalese have known for centuries. Ashwagandha possesses adaptogenic properties, enabling the body to combat stress. It's also hailed for its potential in boosting immunity, enhancing cognitive functions, and even combating the effects of aging.

Furthermore, preliminary research points towards its efficacy in regulating blood sugar levels, and its potential anti-cancer properties are also under investigation.

Balancing Benefits with Awareness

However, like all potent remedies, Ashwagandha is not without its caveats. While generally safe for most, overconsumption or inappropriate intake can lead to side effects. Some individuals might experience upset stomachs, diarrhea, or even allergic reactions.

Pregnant and nursing women are advised to abstain, given the lack of comprehensive studies on its effects during pregnancy. Additionally, those on medication for thyroid conditions should exercise caution, as Ashwagandha might amplify the effects of the drugs.

Blending Narratives: Ashwagandha Meets Other Herbs

The world of herbal teas is vast, and often, it's in the blending that magic happens. Ashwagandha, with its distinct profile, can create harmonious symphonies or discordant notes, depending on its tea partners.

When paired with calming herbs like lavender or chamomile, Ashwagandha's stress-relieving properties are enhanced. Such blends are particularly popular among those seeking solace from the frenzied pace of modern life.

However, blending it with stimulants like green tea or ginseng might attenuate its calming effects, creating a blend that's more invigorating than soothing.

In essence, the blending is an art, a dialogue between herbs, and the narrative changes with each combination.

In the Shadow of the Himalayas: Concluding Thoughts

In Nepal, amidst the echoing chants, the fluttering prayer flags, and the enduring spirit of its people, Ashwagandha has carved its legacy – one that is both ancient and ever-relevant.

From the monastic chambers to the bustling streets of Kathmandu, its presence is felt, revered, and celebrated. In a country that stands as a bridge between the past and the present, Ashwagandha serves as a reminder that sometimes, the answers to the future lie buried in the roots of the past.

Schisandra - A Quintet of Taste

Schisandra Chinensis: An Ode to Complexity

From the dense forests of Northern China and Eastern Russia, an unassuming red berry stands as a testament to nature's paradoxes. Its name, Schisandra Chinensis, might sound exotic, but the myriad tales it carries are universal in their appeal.

As you split open the intricate layers of this berry, it's not just a story of herbal alchemy that unravels, but also of civilizations, migrations, and timeless human pursuits.

The Etymological Ensemble

The term 'Schisandra' traces its lineage to ancient Greek – 'Schizo' means to split, and 'Andra' stands for man, reflecting perhaps the berry's appearance or its multifaceted nature.

But names, as any historian or linguist will attest, carry more than mere descriptions. They're markers of interactions, of cultures brushing against each other, of knowledge transfer, and of shared aspirations. Schisandra, in its etymology, captures this essence.

The Aromatic Aria

Even before one indulges in the taste of the Schisandra tea, the aroma envelopes the senses. It's not a singular note but a cascade. The immediate scent is reminiscent of a forest after a drizzle – earthy, fresh, with an undertone of warmth. As the steam rises, there's a hint of citrus, perhaps an echo of its sour taste, combined with a subtle woodiness.

A Quintet of Tastes

Schisandra is a riddle. How can something be simultaneously sour, sweet, salty, bitter, and pungent? And yet, as one sips the tea made from its berries, each taste makes its presence felt, not clashing but harmonizing.

The initial contact on the palate is sour, evoking memories of wild berries. Just as quickly, there's a shift. The sweetness emerges, not cloying but gentle, reminiscent of ripe fruits. As it courses through the mouth, the salty notes rise, followed by the defining bitterness, cutting through the preceding tastes. And just when one believes the experience is complete, the pungency kicks in, leaving a warming sensation.

It's not merely a beverage but an experience, a sensory journey that offers a glimpse into the vast terrains where Schisandra grows.

Journey to Origins: Where Earth Meets Sky

To truly understand Schisandra, one must journey back, not just in time but in space, to the vast expanses of

Northern China and the taigas of Eastern Russia. Here, in the dense forests, where the winters are harsh and the summers fleeting, Schisandra Chinensis finds its home.

But why here? Any botanist will confirm that plants, like civilizations, are products of their environment. The extreme climates perhaps necessitated the development of these multiple tastes, each a defense mechanism, each a survival strategy. The sourness to deter herbivores, the sweetness to attract birds for seed dispersal, the saltiness from the minerals in the soil, the bitterness to combat insects, and the pungency, a final line of defense against microbial attacks.

Schisandra and Civilization: An Intertwined Tale

No herbal story is complete without the people who discovered, cherished, and propagated it. And in Schisandra's case, it's the ancient Chinese and the native tribes of Eastern Russia who play the protagonists.

In ancient Chinese texts, Schisandra was often referred to as the 'five flavor berry'. It was not merely consumed but revered, finding mentions in medicinal treatises and spiritual texts. Its multifaceted taste was seen as a representation of life's complexities.

In Eastern Russia, Schisandra was more than just a berry; it was a beacon of hope. In the biting cold, when the landscape was draped in a blanket of white, and life seemed to come to a standstill, Schisandra berries offered sustenance, energy, and warmth. The native tribes had their own tales, of warriors consuming Schisandra tea before heading into battles, of shamans using it to connect with the spiritual realm, and of healers prescribing it for ailments ranging from fatigue to digestive issues.

The Vast Russian Expanse

To comprehend the bond between Schisandra and Russia is to plunge deep into the heart of Russian civilization. A vast, sprawling terrain, Russia is a complex tapestry of stories, climates, and souls. Amidst its icy tundras and dense forests, the Russian spirit has found sustenance in nature's bounty. Schisandra is one such gift from the land.

Siberia: The Cradle of Schisandra

Russia is more than just Moscow's gilded domes or St. Petersburg's grand canals. Beyond the urban centers lies Siberia, the heartland of Schisandra. This vast, often inhospitable territory, is where our story takes root.

Life in Siberia has never been easy. The land, while abundant, is also challenging. For the ancient tribes of Siberia, survival depended on understanding and harnessing the environment. And in the deep forests, Schisandra stood as a beacon of resilience.

Tea Time in Taiga

Long before Schisandra became a global sensation, it was the secret of the Siberian Taiga. Ancient tribes, facing the fury of biting winters and fleeting summers, turned to the 'five-flavored berry'. But it wasn't just for sustenance; Schisandra became a symbol.

Imagine a frigid evening, the world blanketed in snow. The night is young, and the tribes gather around a roaring fire. And amidst shared tales and songs, Schisandra tea is brewed. It wasn't just a beverage; it was an experience, a shared moment, a bond forged between man and nature.

Cultural and Spiritual Significance

In the annals of Russian folklore, Schisandra found its place not just as a plant but as a potent symbol. With its five distinct flavors, the berry epitomized life's ebb and flow. The sweetness was joy, the bitterness was sorrow, the saltiness embodied life's surprises, sourness spoke of challenges, and the pungent kick was the spirit's indomitable will.

It wasn't unusual for shamans to employ Schisandra in their rituals, invoking the spirit of the Taiga. It was believed that consuming Schisandra tea helped bridge the gap between the earthly realm and the spiritual world.

Modern Uses and Rediscovery

As centuries passed and Russia morphed from Tsarist empires to Soviet states and into the modern Federation, Schisandra's tale also evolved. With globalization, the world became a smaller place, and Schisandra found itself on international shelves. But for the Russians, it was a rediscovery of sorts.

Today, Schisandra is celebrated for its adaptogenic properties. In a world characterized by stress, hustle, and constant movement, Schisandra offers a moment of balance. Modern research has shed light on its potential benefits, including enhanced cognitive functions, combating fatigue, and even aiding liver health.

Of Blends and Synergies

Tea, in many ways, is a reflection of life. Just as individuals thrive in the company, certain herbs amplify their benefits when paired with others. Schisandra, with its multifaceted flavor profile, offers a unique blending opportunity.

Imagine pairing the sweet-sour notes of Schisandra with the mellow warmth of chamomile or the freshness of mint. Such blends aren't just gustatory delights but also potential health elixirs. However, like any blend, the balance is crucial, ensuring one herb doesn't overshadow the other.

A Note of Caution

Nature, while benevolent, also comes with caveats. Schisandra, for all its glory, isn't exempt. Consuming the tea in moderation is advisable. Overindulgence might lead to heartburn or digestive discomfort in some individuals. As always, pregnant or breastfeeding women and individuals on medications should consult with healthcare professionals before including Schisandra in their regimen.

The Russian Soul: Schisandra's Final Ode

To speak of Schisandra is to embark on a journey across time, terrains, and traditions. In its flavors, one discerns the complexities of the Russian spirit – the joys, the sorrows, the resilience, and the indomitable will. In the modern age, while the contexts have changed, the essence remains. Schisandra isn't just a berry or a tea; it's a fragment of Russia, a tale brewed over millennia.

In the heart of Siberia, as the sun dips below the horizon and the world plunges into twilight, a pot of Schisandra tea simmers, wafting aromas that are as much a promise as they are a memory. And in that moment, the past, present, and future converge, celebrating the timeless dance of man, nature, and history.

Kava - The Elixir of Oceania

Kava whispers, in flavors and scent,
A message of calm, nature's intent.
Plant, aroma, and taste, all in line,
A sip of serenity, time after time.

Kava's Green Majesty

Central to many a Polynesian tale stands the kava plant, *Piper methysticum*, its heart-shaped leaves stretching towards the vast Pacific skies, roots digging deep into the history of the islands. These roots, thick and knotted, carry within them an essence, a spirit, that has captivated the people of Oceania for millennia.

Origins and Etymology: Binding Names and Lands

Etymology often serves as a looking glass into history, and with kava, the journey is no less intriguing. The term 'kava' stems from the Tongan word 'kava', which directly translates to 'bitter'. But kava, in its essence, is anything but simply bitter. It's a complex blend of earthy, peppery notes with a hint of the sea, capturing the very spirit of Oceania.

As for the plant's scientific name, *Piper methysticum*, it echoes the age-old knowledge of the Polynesians. Translated from Latin, it means "intoxicating pepper". The 'pepper' part, *Piper*, is a nod to its place in the pepper family, while 'methysticum' speaks to its effects.

A Symphony of Aromas and Tastes

To describe kava's aroma is to paint a tapestry of the Pacific islands themselves. It's the scent of damp earth after a tropical rain, the saltiness of the sea breeze, and a hint of peppery spice that teases and lingers. It's an aroma that, once known, is never forgotten – instantly recognizable and deeply evocative.

The taste, however, is where kava truly weaves its magic. Earthy and strong, the first sip might catch one off-guard. It's robust, reminiscent of the raw power of the Pacific waves. But as it washes over the palate, there's a subtle numbing, a gentle peppery tang, and a finish that's as serene as a Polynesian lagoon.

Decoding Kava's Soul

The taste and aroma of kava might be captivating, but they are but the surface of a deep ocean of history and culture. To truly understand kava is to delve deep, to immerse oneself in the stories, traditions, and rituals of the Pacific islands.

Polynesia: Navigators of the Vast Pacific

Before one delves into the heart of kava, it is paramount to understand the soul of its people, the Polynesians. The vastness of the Pacific Ocean with its sprawling islands and archipelagos has, for millennia, been the realm of the Polynesians. These weren't just waters and islands; they were pathways, stories, homes. The Polynesians weren't just sailors; they were master navigators, charting courses through stars, winds, and waves, connecting dots in an oceanic expanse with canoes and oral tales.

Yet, their physical journeys on the vast blue were complemented by spiritual voyages, many times fueled by the enigmatic kava.

The Kava Ceremony: More Than a Drink

To an outsider, kava might merely seem like a brew, albeit a potent one. But in Polynesia, it is a bridge – between the past and the present, the mortal and the divine.

The traditional kava ceremony is a tapestry of rituals. The setting is typically a 'malae' or a ceremonial ground. In the center stands the 'tanoa' or kava bowl, carved intricately, telling tales as old as time. Men, often the village elders, sit around it in a circle, symbolizing unity and continuity.

The preparation itself is a dance of hands and rhythms. Roots are cleaned, ground, and then mixed with water, all the while ensuring the age-old techniques are maintained. The resulting liquid, grayish and thick, is then strained through the fibers of the sun-dried 'fau' tree bark or coconut husks, ensuring a smooth blend.

But the act of drinking is where the ceremony truly unfolds. The cup used, usually half a coconut shell, is passed with both hands - a gesture of respect and unity. Before sipping, one would say "Bula" – a term that encapsulates life and health.

It's an experience that transcends the physical realm. It's an act of remembering ancestors, connecting with the gods, and grounding oneself in the present.

A Symbol of Unity and Status

In Polynesian culture, kava wasn't merely a drink; it was a symbol. For leaders and chiefs, sharing kava was a way to solidify alliances, broker peace, or merely re-affirm friendships. Its consumption was, at times, restricted to the noble classes, making it not just a spiritual conduit but also a marker of status.

The Modern Renaissance of Kava

With the tides of time, the world evolved, and so did the place of kava in it. Today, kava bars or 'nakamals' are becoming increasingly popular across the globe, far beyond the sandy shores of Polynesia. Here, in dimly lit spaces with mellow music, people gather not for the high of alcohol but for the calming embrace of kava.

Modern research sheds light on what Polynesians have known for centuries: kava's potential benefits. It's been found to have anxiolytic effects, potentially aiding those grappling with anxiety disorders. Some studies suggest it might help in sleep induction, given its calming properties.

Cautionary Tales: The Double-Edged Sword

Yet, as with many potent brews, kava isn't without its shadows. Chronic, heavy consumption has been linked with liver issues. Some cases, though rare, have even reported hepatitis, cirrhosis, and liver failure. Furthermore, it can potentially interact with medications, particularly those that act on the liver.

The traditional Polynesian preparation methods, which focus on the root, tend to be safer. It's the inclusion of other plant parts and non-traditional preparations that often lead to complications.

Kava's Dance with Other Herbs

In the realm of herbal concoctions, combining different elements can either be harmonious or clash terribly. With kava, this dance is intricate. Its sedative effects mean it can amplify the effects of other calming herbs like valerian or chamomile. But combine it with stimulants, and the mixture can be jarring. The key is balance and knowledge.

Polynesia, with its vast skies, shimmering waters, and the haunting call of distant horizons, has given the world many gifts. But few are as enigmatic, as soulful, as the kava. In its bitter taste lies the salt of the ocean, in its calming embrace, the serenity of a Pacific night, and in its depth, the very soul of a civilization. Through kava, one doesn't just drink; one remembers, feels, and transcends.

Passionflower – Emissary of Dreams

Soft on the tongue, hints of earthy grace,
Passionflower's touch, a gentle embrace.
Mildly sweet, with an undertone light,
Like stars shimmering, in the heart of the night.

Passionflower: Nature's Ornate Conception

Delicately complex, the Passionflower, or *Passiflora*, is nature's ode to intricacy. A blossom that seems to have been designed with great deliberation and an artist's meticulousness, it is an explosion of petals, filaments, and tendrils. Every segment of this flower tells a tale, and together, they compose an exquisite symphony of nature.

But why the name 'Passion' for this ethereal flower? Some might imagine it stems from its seductive beauty, a passion it ignites in the beholder's heart. But the tale winds back to the early Spanish colonists of South America, who saw in its structure the symbols of the Passion of Christ. The flower's ten petals and sepals were likened to the apostles, its corona filaments to Christ's crown of thorns, and its tendrils to the whips.

The Origins: Tracing the Threads of Time

While Europe named it, the Passionflower's story began much earlier and in a world far removed from the Iberian Peninsula. The heart of the Amazon rainforest, with its ceaseless cacophony of life, was where the Passionflower first spread its tendrils.

Here, amidst the dense foliage, the dappled sunlight, and the rhythmic chants of myriad creatures, the *Passiflora* thrived, weaving its way through the trees, often reaching for the heavens.

Etymology: A Religious Resonance

As aforementioned, the term 'Passionflower' is steeped in Christian symbolism. Coined by Spanish Christian missionaries, the name was derived from the Latin word 'passio', meaning suffering, and 'flos', meaning flower. They believed the flower was a divine sign, representing the last days of Jesus Christ, making it not just a botanical wonder but also a spiritual emblem.

The Sensory Experience: Aroma and Taste

To approach the Passionflower is to be embraced by an aroma that's both subtle and profound. It doesn't overwhelm; it beckons. A gentle sweetness, with earthy undertones, reminiscent of the dense forest grounds from which it emerges.

When transformed into a tea, the Passionflower carries its elegance forth. The brew is a pale gold, and as it touches the palate, it's almost like a whispered lullaby. Mildly grassy with hints of floral sweetness, it's a tea that doesn't shout its presence. Instead, it gently envelopes, soothes, and caresses.

A Symphony of the Forest: Indigenous Tribes of the Amazon

The vast expanse of the Amazon rainforest, with its green cathedral canopies and the relentless chatter of life, has for millennia been home to a plethora of indigenous tribes. These tribes, each unique, have together painted a rich tapestry of culture, tradition, and an intimacy with nature that's nearly unparalleled. Their knowledge of the forest, the flora, and the fauna, is not just about survival; it's a profound understanding, a deep conversation, passed down generations.

From Leaf to Cup: The Ritualistic Brewing

The Amazon tribes, such as the Yanomami, the Kayapo, and the Tupi, amongst others, have been attuned to the bounties of their environment. To them, the Passionflower wasn't just another exotic bloom but a medicinal treasure. Traditionally, leaves and stems of the plant were carefully selected, dried in the shade of the enormous rainforest trees, and then, when the moment was right, brewed into a tea.

Yet, it was never merely about the act of brewing. It was ritualistic, almost a form of meditation. Every step, from selecting the right leaves to the final sip, was performed with reverence, underscoring their deep bond with nature.

A Spiritual Elixir? The Deeper Layers

To these tribes, every element of the rainforest, from the mightiest jaguar to the smallest flower, held significance. The Passionflower was no different. While we, with our modern lens, may perceive it as a relaxation agent, for these tribes, it was more profound.

Whispers in the tribe spoke of the flower as a spiritual conduit. The tea, when consumed in the right setting, often under the guidance of a shaman, was believed to bridge the earthly and the ethereal, providing glimpses into one's inner self, dreams, and even prophetic visions.

Modern Embrace: The Therapeutic Treasure

As the world woke up to the wonders of the Amazon, the Passionflower too found itself in the limelight. Today, the realms of alternative medicine and even mainstream pharmacology recognize the flower's calming properties.

Passionflower tea, in our frenetic modern world, serves as an anchor. Its mild sedative effects are sought after for anxiety relief, managing insomnia, and even as an aid against opioid withdrawal. Moreover, studies have shown that it can augment levels of gamma-aminobutyric acid (GABA) in the brain, a compound that lowers brain activity, thereby helping one relax.

Potential Side Effects

While predominantly safe, especially when consumed in moderation, some may experience dizziness, confusion, or atypical coordination. It's also worth noting that in very high doses, it can lead to increased heart rate or erratic heartbeat patterns.

Moreover, pregnant or breastfeeding women are generally advised to refrain from consuming Passionflower, primarily due to insufficient research in this area.

Mingling with Other Brews: Interactions and Synergies

Tea blends are a testament to our never-ending quest for the perfect taste or therapeutic effect. Passionflower, with its mild taste profile and calming properties, is often blended with other herbs. When mixed with chamomile or valerian root, the sedative effect is often enhanced, creating a potent brew for relaxation or sleep.

However, one must tread with caution. Combining Passionflower with other sedative herbs or medications can lead to an exaggerated response, and its interaction with anticoagulants is still a subject of study.

Amidst the shadows of the Amazon, where every rustle tells a story and every dawn brings a renewed symphony of life, the Passionflower has carved its own legend. From the spiritual rituals of the indigenous tribes to the teacups of the modern anxious world, its journey has been profound.

To truly appreciate the Passionflower is to recognize its dual legacy: the ancient wisdom of the Amazon tribes and the scientific validations of today. In this duality lies its magic – rooted in tradition, yet relevant in modernity. It's not just a tea; it's a testament to the timeless dance of nature and culture.

Hawthorn – Guardian of The Heart

Rich and robust, a flavor profound,
Hawthorn's essence, in every round.
Hints of berries, and autumn's embrace,
A hearty sip, nature's grace.

From Thorned Bough to Steaming Brew

The Hawthorn tree, bearing its vibrant berries and boasting a rich, robust history, stands like a sentinel across landscapes, its boughs whispering secrets from the past. The tree itself, belonging to the genus *Crataegus*, is a vision of contrasts - delicate blossoms and sharp thorns, embodying the juxtapositions of life itself.

Origins & Etymology: Tracing Roots

The term 'Hawthorn' is derived from the Old English 'hagathorn', where 'haga' means 'hedge'. Indeed, this tree was frequently used as hedging in agricultural landscapes. But the name is not just an empty label; it's emblematic of the tree's place in the landscape and culture, an enduring symbol of boundaries, both physical and metaphysical.

The etymology offers a portal into understanding not just the plant, but the societies that named and utilized it. It's a hint that the tree was integral, not just to the landscape, but also to the fabric of the communities that lived alongside it.

A Symphony of Senses: Aroma & Taste

To describe the aroma of Hawthorn tea is to narrate a story. The first whiff is subtly floral, reminiscent of late spring mornings when the first blossoms start to open. But as you inhale deeply, there's an underlying earthiness, grounding the ethereal floral notes, tethering them to the rich, loamy soils where the tree sinks its roots.

And then, the taste. It begins with a mellow sweetness, almost berry-like, but more complex. This initial sweetness gives way to a mild tang, reminiscent of the wild, windswept landscapes the Hawthorn often calls home. It's a taste that's both refreshing and haunting, a reminder of nature's duality.

The Hawthorn Beyond the Tea

While this chapter might find its culmination in a steaming cup of Hawthorn tea, the tree's history is not merely confined to its culinary uses. The Hawthorn, with its stark thorns and blossoms, has been symbolic in numerous cultures, representing everything from hope and merriment to warnings and barriers.

The Emerald Isle's Ethos

Before one dives into the Celtic weave of tales surrounding the Hawthorn, it's crucial to paint a portrait of the civilization that held it so dear. Ireland, an island sequestered in the North Atlantic, is far more than its postcard panorama of undulating green landscapes. It is a land whose heart beats in time with ancient drumbeats, a land crisscrossed with ley lines of legends and traditions.

The Irish have long held a unique kinship with the land. Their identity, songs, and stories are carved from the very soil they tread upon. A fertile ground for tales of faeries and spirits, this civilization has ever been in intimate dialogue with nature, seeking meanings, messages, and miracles in its embrace.

The Whisper of Faeries and the Hawthorn Tree

In the Irish consciousness, the Hawthorn occupies a space both mundane and mystical. On one hand, it's a hedge plant, demarcating territories and farms. But as night falls and the world blurs at the edges, the Hawthorn transforms.

It was widely believed among the Irish that Hawthorn trees, especially those standing alone, were the meeting points for the Aos Sí, the faeries. They were thus known as 'Faerie trees'. Disturbing such a tree, be it for its wood or to clear land, was considered not just inauspicious but a direct affront to the fae folk, possibly leading to dire consequences.

While one might see such beliefs as mere superstition, they underscore the Irish way of harmonious living with nature, where every tree and stone is imbued with spirit and significance.

From Hedgerows to Hearth: The Hawthorn Brew

Given the spiritual significance of the Hawthorn, it's hardly surprising that it made its way into the daily lives of the Irish. Though its ethereal associates might have dissuaded casual plucking, under proper rites and respect, the Hawthorn offered its blessings in the form of tea.

Hawthorn tea, often brewed from the leaves and flowers, was an age-old remedy. Folk healers and wise women would often prescribe it for heart ailments. But beyond the physical, it was also believed to be a tonic for the emotional heart, mending broken spirits and soothing turbulent emotions.

Modern Elixirs: The Hawthorn in Contemporary Wellness

Time has done little to diminish the Hawthorn's allure. Modern herbalists continue to champion its benefits, albeit with the backing of scientific research. Its antioxidant properties, coupled with its ability to regulate blood pressure and promote cardiovascular health, make it a favored choice in today's holistic health circles.

But the Hawthorn offers more than mere physical benefits. In an age characterized by emotional turbulence and stress, many find solace in its calming properties, echoing the age-old Irish belief of its power over the heart's matters.

A Word of Caution: The Tea's Two Edges

Like all potent remedies, the Hawthorn's brew is not without its caveats. While generally considered safe, overconsumption can lead to dizziness, nausea, and digestive troubles. Those on heart medications should approach with caution, as the tea can amplify or interfere with the drugs' effects.

Blending Traditions: Hawthorn's Dance with Other Herbs

Hawthorn's versatile nature allows it to gracefully entwine with other herbal notes. When paired with Ginkgo, for instance, the duo amplifies cardiovascular benefits. With calming Chamomile, it becomes a bedtime brew, promoting both heart health and restful sleep.

Yet, it's essential to approach these blends with knowledge. Pairing Hawthorn with too many diuretic herbs might exacerbate its effects, leading to potential complications.

Conclusion: The Hawthorn's Legacy

In the winding paths of history, as civilizations rise and fall, certain constants endure. For Ireland, the Hawthorn stands as a testament to its age-old romance with nature, a symbol of its deep-rooted traditions and beliefs.

As modernity encroaches, and skyscrapers threaten to overshadow ancient groves, the story of the Hawthorn serves as a poignant reminder. It beckons us to remember, respect, and revere the delicate dance between man and nature, to find the magic in the mundane, and to seek solace in the arms of age-old trees and traditions.

St. John's Wort – The Witches' Bane

Tiny yellow blooms, amidst green so bright,
St. John's Wort stands, bathed in light.
Nature's remedy, for souls that yearn,
Healing hearts, at every turn.

A Plant of Light in Nature's Green

When one wanders through European meadows during midsummer, they might be greeted by a sea of yellow — golden petals reflecting the sun's brilliance. These are the flowers of Hypericum perforatum, commonly known as St. John's Wort. Its name translates to "over an apparition," hinting at its ancient association with dispelling evil spirits. Indeed, much of the plant's lore revolves around protection and light, concepts eternally intertwined in the human psyche.

Upon close examination, this perennial herb, reaching up to 90 cm in height, exhibits translucent dots on its leaves. When crushed, these spots release a crimson oil, reminiscent of the blood of St. John the Baptist, for whom the plant is named. The red pigment is hypericin, a compound that has long fascinated and remains a subject of research to this day.

Etymology: The Naming of a Savior Herb

The name 'St. John's Wort' is no accidental moniker. The appellation 'wort' is an Old English term meaning 'plant' or 'herb'. But why St. John? The herb traditionally blooms around the time of the Feast of St. John the Baptist on June 24th. Its bright yellow flowers were said to represent the halo of St. John, and its red pigment, his martyrdom. But there's more depth to this nomenclature, a depth that delves into the psyche of the civilizations that revered it.

Aroma and Taste: The Sensory Experience

Much like its bright appearance, St. John's Wort's aroma can be described as bittersweet, with a woody undertone, evoking memories of a summer's day. A hint of a floral note, like that of its yellow blossoms, often teases the olfactory senses. When steeped into tea, it carries a mild, earthy flavor, with a subtle sweetness, reminiscent of sun-warmed hay fields. Unlike more potent herbal brews, its gentleness on the palate makes it a favored choice for many.

Deep Roots in Ancient Soil

To understand St. John's Wort, we must traverse the corridors of time to ancient Greece. The Greeks, with their pantheon of gods and expansive pharmacopeia, recognized the plant's value. Dioscorides and Hippocrates, towering figures in ancient medicine, documented its use. But its history doesn't start or end there.

The ancient Druids, predating Christian influence, considered it a sacred herb, using it in their midsummer festivals. As Christianity spread, these pagan practices were absorbed and adapted, with St. John's Wort becoming associated with St. John the Baptist.

In the subsequent centuries, its use and significance evolved, shifting from spiritual to more medicinal applications, yet always retaining an aura of mystery and reverence.

Whispers of the Holy Roman Empire

To grasp the profound influence of St. John's Wort in the medieval German landscape, we must first meander through the cobblestone streets of the Holy Roman Empire. The Empire, a complex conglomeration of territories in central Europe, was a cauldron of politics, faith, and evolving thought. Yet, amidst this ever-changing political and religious canvas, one constant remained - the undying bond of its people with nature, and their reliance on herbal remedies.

The Medieval German Household: An Apothecary Within

Before delving into the bond between the Germans and St. John's Wort, it's pivotal to understand the quintessential medieval German household. More often than not, it was equipped with a 'Hausapotheke' or home pharmacy. This collection was not merely a compendium of dried herbs; it was an ancestral legacy passed down with great reverence.

In these assortments, St. John's Wort occupied a place of honor. Known as 'Johanniskraut' in German, echoing St. John the Baptist, the herb's presence was both protective and curative.

St. John's Eve: Of Fires and Festivities

The summer solstice, and particularly St. John's Eve, was an occasion of great merriment and significance. As dusk descended, bonfires dotted the German landscape. These flames, symbolizing the sun at its zenith, served dual purposes: a celebration of light and a ward against malevolent spirits. Into these fires, bunches of St. John's Wort were thrown. The resulting flames, tinged with a unique hue, were believed to possess protective powers.

For the common folk, this was more than mere festivity. It was a fusion of their pagan roots with adopted Christian practices. In this confluence, St. John's Wort wasn't just a herb; it was a beacon of hope, a shield against darkness, both literal and metaphorical. Homes would often find their doorways graced with the herb, not just as a celebration of midsummer but as a talisman against the darkness, a sentinel against the supernatural.

Witches, those enigmatic beings often misunderstood and maligned, were believed to be repelled by the herb. It's a curious juxtaposition: an era where the same nature that provided remedies also hid unseen menaces. And in this world, where the boundaries between the natural and supernatural were porous, St. John's Wort stood as a shield.

Medicinal Elixirs and Potions: St. John's Wort in Healing

Beyond the mystical, the practical applications of Johanniskraut were manifold. Medieval German texts, echoing the wisdom of monks and healers, often sang praises of its remedial virtues. Infusions of the herb, taken as tea, were popular for alleviating melancholia, what we understand today as depression. Topical applications, often as balms or oils, promised relief from burns, wounds, and neuralgic pains.

Spirituality and Symbolism

To the devout, the herb's blooming around St. John's feast day wasn't mere coincidence. It was Divine providence. Its golden flowers were symbolic of the light of St. John, and the red pigment was a somber reminder of his sacrifice. In a world where the veil between the sacred and the profane was gossamer thin, St. John's Wort was a tangible link to the Divine.

Modern Revelations and Resonances

Centuries have passed since the medieval era, but St. John's Wort's allure hasn't waned. Modern science, with its tools and tenacity, has validated what the Germans instinctively knew. The herb indeed possesses compounds, notably hypericin and hyperforin, that influence mood. Today, it's recognized as a natural antidepressant, offering solace to many.

Caveats and Interactions

Yet, as with all potent remedies, St. John's Wort isn't without its cautions. While the medieval Germans imbibed their brews with faith, our contemporary understanding urges moderation. The herb can potentiate the effects of certain medications, including antidepressants. Moreover, it can heighten sensitivity to sunlight in some.

Its interaction with other herbal teas is intricate. When blended with calming herbs like chamomile, the result is often a synergistic soothe. However, combined with stimulants like green tea, one must tread with caution.

Conclusion: Legacy of Light

From the medieval meadows to modern mugs, St. John's Wort remains a luminary. The German people, with their intrinsic bond with nature, recognized and revered its power. Today, as we sip its brew, we aren't just consuming a tea; we're imbibing a legacy — a legacy of hope, healing, and the undying human spirit.

Jasmine Tea - The Fragrant Soul of Asia

Floral notes, softly they play,
On the tongue, in a ballet.
Delicate hints of springtime's grace,
Every sip, an embrace.

From Garden to Goblet: The Plant Behind the Potion

Jasmine's botanical tale is as enchanting as its aroma. It belongs to the *Oleaceae* family, a family that also graciously gives us the olive. Among the 200 species, it's primarily the common jasmine (*Jasminum officinale*) and the Sampaguita (*Jasminum sambac*) that are courted for tea. Delicate white blossoms, often with a slight pinkish hue, are plucked under the cloak of dusk, as that's when they are most fragrant. These blossoms, in their unassuming beauty, hold within them an aroma that has beguiled emperors and poets alike.

Whence Came the Jasmine? A Journey of Origins

Tracing the jasmine's footprints lands us primarily in the cradle of ancient Persia, though its tendrils extend to various corners of Asia. Its etymology, like a fragrant breeze, wafted through Latin, where 'jasminum' was derived from the Persian 'yasamen'. The latter, echoing the soft, gentle quality of the aroma, means a 'gift from God'.

Yet, how did this Persian gem traverse to China and then meld with tea? The silken threads of history, as intricate as the famed Silk Road, weave tales of trade, diplomacy, and cultural exchange. By the Tang Dynasty, jasmine had firmly rooted itself in the Chinese landscape. However, its union with tea – that was a serendipitous chapter yet to be written.

A Symphony of Scents: The Aroma and Taste of Jasmine Tea

Imagine, for a moment, a tranquil garden bathed in moonlight. As crickets orchestrate their nightly symphonies, jasmine blossoms bloom, releasing their pent-up fragrance. This very tableau is captured in every cup of jasmine tea. The aroma is undeniably floral, but with a depth and complexity that's hard to define. It hints at sweetness, at warmth, and at a certain ethereal quality that is quintessentially jasmine.

The taste? It's a harmonious blend of the mild vegetal notes of green tea (most commonly used for jasmine tea) and the unmistakable heady fragrance of jasmine. There's an initial sweetness, which then gives way to a slightly astringent finish, making every sip an intricate dance of flavors.

Melding Petals with Leaves: The Craft of Jasmine Tea

The creation of jasmine tea is an art form, a testament to human ingenuity and patience. After the tea leaves, typically green or white, are harvested, they undergo minimal processing. These semi-processed leaves are then stored until late summer when jasmine blossoms are in their fragrant prime.

Once plucked, the blossoms are stored in a cool place until nightfall. Under the shroud of darkness, when the flowers commence their aromatic bloom, they are layered with tea leaves. This is no haphazard layering, but a meticulous process, often done by hand. As dawn approaches, the flowers, having shared their fragrance with the tea, are removed. This nocturnal dance is repeated multiple times, sometimes up to seven nights, until the tea leaves are suffused with the fragrance.

Vietnam: The Land of Ascending Dragons

Vietnam, with its lush green valleys and long serpentine coast, whispers tales of legendary dragons and ancient spirits. For thousands of years, the resilient Vietnamese have toiled their land, battled invaders, and woven a rich tapestry of culture and tradition. They've been rice cultivators, fearless warriors, poetic dreamers, and avid tea drinkers.

It is essential to understand that Vietnam isn't just a singular entity but a mosaic of ethnicities, beliefs, and traditions. From the Hmong tribes of the northern mountains to the Khmer influences in the Mekong Delta, the country is a vibrant puzzle of histories and influences.

Jasmine Tea in Vietnam: More than a Sip

In a nation where tea-drinking is as natural as breathing, the advent of jasmine tea adds another layer to the country's complex beverage tapestry. To the Vietnamese, drinking tea is a ritual, a communal event, and a moment of reflection. Enter jasmine tea, with its intoxicating aroma and delicate taste, and it's no wonder that it found a favored spot in the Vietnamese tea repertoire.

But how did jasmine, primarily an import from Persia, make its aromatic mark on Vietnamese tea culture? As history would have it, Vietnam's close geographical and cultural proximity to China, especially the southern provinces, played a role. The interchange of goods, ideas, and agricultural practices between these neighboring giants facilitated the jasmine plant's journey to Vietnam.

Cultural and Spiritual Significance

Under the Tenderness of Moonlight

To truly grasp the spiritual gravity of jasmine tea in Vietnam, one must first fathom the Vietnamese Moon Festival or *Tết Trung Thu*. A festival that celebrates the biggest and brightest of lunar displays, it's a time for family, for lanterns, and for reflection.

As lanterns illuminate the night, tales of ancient legends are whispered, and here, in this ambient setting, jasmine tea often makes its aromatic appearance. The tea, with its moonlit-white blossoms, serves as an echo of the celestial body above. The Vietnamese believe in harmonizing with nature, and what better way to pay homage to the moon than with a tea that seemingly captures its essence?

An Offering of Fragrance

Jasmine tea also often graces the altars of Vietnamese homes and temples. It's not just a beverage but an offering.

The aroma of the tea is believed to appease and attract benevolent spirits. In a culture where ancestors are revered, a cup of jasmine tea serves as a bridge between the earthly realm and the ethereal.

Modern Uses and the Spectrum of Health Benefits

Though deeply rooted in tradition, the consumption of jasmine tea in contemporary Vietnam isn't just a nod to the past. The modern Vietnamese, living in bustling cities like Ho Chi Minh City or Hanoi, find solace in this fragrant brew.

Cardiovascular Boon: Jasmine tea, particularly when melded with green tea leaves, contains a significant amount of antioxidants. These antioxidants play a pivotal role in reducing LDL cholesterol levels and improving overall heart health.

Stress Relief: The very act of brewing jasmine tea, watching the delicate petals unfurl, coupled with its serene aroma, has a calming effect. The presence of L-theanine amplifies this calming effect, making it an excellent ally against modern-day stress.

Digestive Aid: In Vietnam, meals are often lavish affairs. Jasmine tea, post such meals, aids in digestion. It acts as a gentle carminative, reducing bloating and ensuring smooth digestion.

Potential Side Effects

Like all good things in life, moderation is key. While jasmine tea is a treasure trove of benefits, excessive consumption could lead to:

Sleep Disturbances: The caffeine content, albeit lower than coffee, can cause insomnia if consumed late in the evening.

Allergies: A rare occurrence, but some individuals might be allergic to jasmine and could manifest symptoms like itching or respiratory problems.

Interactions with Other Herbal Teas

In Vietnam, jasmine tea, though perfect in its singularity, sometimes gets blended with other herbal teas. This isn't just a culinary experiment but often has roots in traditional medicine.

Jasmine and Lotus: The combination of jasmine's floral notes with the earthy tones of lotus creates a blend that's both aromatic and grounding. In traditional Vietnamese medicine, this blend is believed to harmonize the mind and body.

Jasmine and Pandan: A blend that's becoming increasingly popular, the sweet grassy notes of pandan complement the heady aroma of jasmine. This mix is not only delicious but is also considered cooling for the body.

Jasmine Tea - Vietnam's Liquid Aria

In Vietnam, jasmine tea isn't a mere beverage. It's an experience, an aromatic journey through the country's valleys and traditions. Through wars, colonizations, and modernizations, jasmine tea has remained, steadfast and fragrant, capturing the very essence of Vietnam in its delicate aroma. A cup of this tea is more than just a drink; it's a liquid aria

Saw Palmetto - The Gentleman's Elixir

Untamed flavors, bold and free,
A dance of wildness and tranquility.
From the land, to the sea's shallow,
Such is the taste of Saw Palmetto.

Saw Palmetto: The Modest Monarch of the Understory

Beneath the towering pines and the stately oaks of the Southeastern United States, the Saw Palmetto (*Serenoa repens*) claims its dominion. Not with the majesty of height, for it is but a humble palm, but with its sheer omnipresence. One can't help but notice the fan-shaped leaves, serrated along the petiole, giving it its evocative name.

At first glance, this palm might seem inconspicuous, even ordinary. But delve deeper, and it's clear that the Saw Palmetto has carved a niche for itself in the annals of botany and human civilization.

From Ancient Earth to Modern Science: Origins and Etymology

An Ancient Survivor

Saw Palmetto, given its current distribution, has ancient roots. Fossils suggest the existence of this palm dating back to millennia. It's a relic of epochs gone by, having witnessed the ebb and flow of ice ages, the migrations of megafauna, and the evolution of its surrounding ecosystem.

Etymological Excursions

The genus name "Serenoa" is a nod to American botanist Sereno Watson. While "repens" reflects its growth habit – creeping, sprawling, and forever expanding. The common name, however, is a descriptor. "Saw" refers to the sharp, tooth-like serrations, and "Palmetto" signifies its kinship with palms. It's a name that's both functional and evocative, hinting at its unique character and appearance.

The Symphony of Scents and Flavors

An Aroma that Speaks of Earth

Crack open a berry of Saw Palmetto, and it tells a tale. The scent is reminiscent of the earth after rain – fresh, raw, and rich. There's a certain pungency, a whisper of the wetlands, the marshes, and the sandy soils from which it springs. The aroma isn't just a sensory experience but a transportive one, connecting us to the very lands the Seminoles once roamed.

A Taste Rooted in Tradition

To describe the flavor of Saw Palmetto tea is to narrate a story of complexities. There's a certain bitterness, yes, but also an underlying sweetness, subtle and easily missed. Some might detect a hint of pepper, a touch of green, or a whisper of the forest. It's a tea that requires contemplation, urging the drinker to pause, reflect, and uncover its layers.

The Seminole: A People Undefined by Conquest
From Creek Confederacy to Florida's Swamps

The Seminole story is as resilient and untamed as the saw palmettos they used. Originating from the Creek Confederacy, the Seminole sought refuge in Florida's wilds, escaping the encroaching European settlers. Florida wasn't just an escape but a haven, a place where their spirit could resonate with the land. Here, among the mangroves, marshes, and pinelands, they melded with other tribes, birthing a unique culture.

The Unconquered: Resistance and Identity

The Seminoles, often termed the "Unconquered People", aren't just defined by their resistance to European settlers and the U.S. government but also by their unwavering spirit. Three Seminole Wars couldn't break them, nor could attempts at assimilation. Their identity was and remains as much a product of their spirited resistance as their integration with Florida's wild environment.

The Sacred Brew: Saw Palmetto in the Seminole Life
Nourishment from the Land

For the Seminole, the saw palmetto was more than just vegetation; it was sustenance, both physical and spiritual. The berries were an essential food source, and the fronds provided shelter, but it was the tea that connected them to the land spiritually.

As with many indigenous communities, the Seminole believed in the harmony of body and environment. Saw palmetto tea, with its earthy aroma and complex taste, was emblematic of this belief. It wasn't merely consumed; it was meditated upon.

Spiritual Symbolism

The preparation and consumption of saw palmetto tea were rituals, spaces where the physical act met the metaphysical. The Seminoles held the view that ailments weren't just physical disturbances but spiritual imbalances. Drinking the tea, which they believed housed the spirit of the land, was a way of realigning one's spirit with the universe.

While no detailed written records exist of these ceremonies, oral traditions speak of chants, dances, and meditative silences accompanying the tea's consumption, each a step in the journey towards spiritual alignment.

From Traditional Brew to Modern Cup: Health Benefits of Saw Palmetto Tea

The Science Behind the Spirituality

Modern science, in its ever-curious quest, has explored the saw palmetto's depths, and the results affirm many of the Seminoles' beliefs.

- **Prostate Health**: Perhaps the most recognized benefit of saw palmetto tea today is its role in maintaining prostate health. The compounds in the tea have been found to reduce symptoms of benign prostatic hyperplasia (BPH).

- **Balancing Hormones**: Saw palmetto can also influence hormone levels, making it useful in conditions like polycystic ovary syndrome (PCOS).

- **Anti-Inflammatory**: The tea possesses anti-inflammatory properties, which could explain its traditional use in soothing digestive or respiratory issues.

Potential Side Effects

As with any remedy, moderation and understanding are key. While saw palmetto tea offers numerous health benefits, it's not without its potential side effects:

- **Digestive Issues**: Some people may experience digestive disturbances, including nausea or diarrhea.

- **Hormonal Imbalance**: Given its impact on hormones, it's crucial to consult with a healthcare provider, especially if one is on hormone therapies or birth control.

- **Drug Interactions**: Saw palmetto might interact with certain medications, including blood thinners and NSAIDs.

Blending Traditions: Interactions with Other Herbal Teas

Saw palmetto tea, with its distinct flavor profile, can be blended with other herbal teas, both enhancing its taste and complementing its effects. However, care must be taken:

- With hormone-regulating teas like **chasteberry**, the combined effects might be too potent, leading to hormonal imbalances.

- Teas with diuretic properties, such as **nettle tea**, might amplify the effects, leading to dehydration if consumed in large quantities.

- On the flip side, blending with **chamomile** or **peppermint** can soothe the digestive system, potentially countering any minor disturbances caused by the saw palmetto.

In Conclusion: An Ode to Resilience, in Leaves and Lives

The tale of saw palmetto tea isn't just about a beverage; it's about a people, their land, and the intimate ties between them. It's a story that spans millennia, from the Seminoles' spirited dances to the modern tea enthusiast's meditative sips. In the heart of this narrative lies a lesson on the harmonious coexistence of nature and culture, and the timeless wisdom indigenous communities offer. As we sip our saw palmetto tea, may we always remember the Seminole spirit, and may we strive to live in harmony with our environment, just as they did.

The Leaf of Legends - Camellia Sinensis

In our journey, we've traversed the gardens of thirty distinct herbal infusions, we've uncovered their secrets, their therapeutic promises, and some of the civilizations that have held them dear. Yet, there remains one tea that stands as a colossus, casting its shadow over all others—Camellia sinensis. It would be an oversight, nay, an omission, not to journey down its rich path. Thus, we now turn our gaze to the stalwarts of tradition: Black, Green, and White tea.

Black Tea

Steeped in tradition, strong and bold,
A tale of empires in every fold.
Whispers of smoke and molten gold,
Awakening senses, stories retold.

Green Tea

Veil of mist and morning's dew,
Emerald essence, a vibrant hue.
Hints of dawn, the day's first line,
Nature's pulse, serenely divine.

White Tea

Ethereal touch, a gentle breeze,
Whispers of petals, nature's tease.
Subtle and soft, it takes its flight,
In delicate sips of purest white.

The Threefold Elixir: Camellia sinensis Unveiled

The Singular Plant: A Bountiful Source

One plant, three distinct teas. Such is the enigmatic prowess of *Camellia sinensis*. Whether you're pouring a robust cup of black tea, a refreshing green, or the delicate white, you're sipping from the leaves of this singular tree. It's not magic but a meticulous alchemy of processing that transforms these leaves into the diverse spectrums of flavor and aroma.

Origins: Tracing the Root of the Leaf

The earliest whispers of *Camellia sinensis* trace back to Yunnan Province in today's China. Legends, perhaps slightly embellished over time, speak of ancient emperors and accidental brews. However, beneath the allure of these tales lies a truth – China was, undoubtedly, the cradle of tea cultivation.

The Etymological Journey: From Cha to Té and Beyond

Language, ever so reflective of trade and cultural exchanges, charts its own narrative of tea's journey.

The Chinese 'Cha'

In its homeland, it was 'cha.' This phonetic lingered in the languages of the nations touched by the Silk Road – Persian, Arabic, and even Russian.

European 'Té'

Europe's introduction to tea, predominantly through maritime routes, coined a different phonetic – té, as the

Portuguese would say. This distinction between 'cha' and 'té' isn't merely linguistic but subtly hints at the geopolitics of trade routes.

Symphony of the Senses: Aroma and Taste

The world of *Camellia sinensis* is vast, and its sensory spectrum, vaster. Processing the leaf is akin to composing music – the same notes, when arranged differently, produce distinct melodies.

Black Tea: The Robust Ballad

Fermented to fullness, black tea sings a bold song. The aroma – at times malty, sometimes smoky, or even fruity – speaks of its journey: from the flush of the leaf to the intricacies of processing. As for its taste, it resonates with the depths of its color: robust, with a satisfying astringency.

Green Tea: The Refreshing Lilt

Untouched by fermentation, green tea retains the youthful exuberance of the leaf. Its aroma, grassy and vegetal, is the scent of spring. On the palate, it dances with a lightness, a delicate balance of sweetness and bitterness.

White Tea: A Gentle Whisper

The least processed of the triad, white tea is subtlety personified. Derived from the young buds, its aroma is faint – floral, with a hint of fruitiness. The taste is a soft echo of its scent, smooth, with a silken sweetness.

A Global Narrative

The tale of black, green, and white tea – from its botanical birth to its aromatic allure – sets the stage for a global odyssey. A simple leaf of *Camellia sinensis* has played muse to emperors, monks, and merchants alike. The legacy of tea is as complex as its flavors, interwoven with commerce, culture, and conquests.

The Eastern Sunrise: The Genesis of Tea Rituals

China's Sacred Sips

The sprawling empire of China, with its vast terrains and dynastic shifts, holds the primordial secrets of tea. The story, as documented in Tang dynasty texts, begins with Emperor Shen Nong's fateful discovery around 2737 BCE. As legend would have it, some stray leaves from a burning tea bush drifted into the emperor's pot of boiling water. And just like that, a refreshing potion was born.

For the Chinese, tea was more than mere sustenance. It was the fabric of their culture. Philosophers and scholars infused it into their teachings; artists and poets captured its essence on canvases and in verses. The famed 'Cha Jing' or 'The Classic of Tea', written by Lu Yu during the Tang dynasty, attests to the deep reverence China held for this brew. It wasn't simply about the taste but the art of preparation, appreciation, and consumption.

Japan's Steeped Traditions

A sip away from China, Japan imbibed the tea culture somewhere around the 8th century. Initially consumed by priests and nobility, it was Eisai, a Buddhist monk, who popularized the health benefits of green tea. His work, 'Kissa Yōjōki' or 'How to Stay Healthy by Drinking Tea', became the cornerstone of Japan's tea traditions.

But Japan did not just adopt; it adapted. The meticulous Japanese tea ceremony or 'Chanoyu' emerged, emphasizing the beauty in every step of tea-making, from whisking matcha to the etiquette of sipping.

The Western Horizon: Tea Takes Europe

Portuguese Pursuits and Dutch Determination

While tales of tea had wafted into European courts, the first serious encounter came via the Portuguese in the 16th century. It was their trade with China that marked Europe's inaugural introduction to this Eastern elixir.

However, it was the Dutch who took the mantle of tea's primary purveyors in Europe. Their merchant ships laden with tea leaves docked at ports, making Amsterdam the continent's early tea capital.

Britain's Brewing Obsession

Yet, it was Britain, an empire upon which the sun never set, that truly became obsessed. By the 17th century, tea was more than an exotic novelty; it was a national fixation. The 'afternoon tea' tradition commenced, an affair that went beyond the beverage, encapsulating a specific time, an array of delicacies, and an entire social ritual.

And as Britain expanded its colonial footprints, so did its thirst for tea. This very obsession paved the way for opium wars, colonial expeditions, and the cultivation of tea in new terrains like India.

From Colonial Cultivations to Global Grails

India's Assam Awakening and Darjeeling Delight

Ironically, while Britain's fervor for tea began with China, it was India that became its largest supplier by the 19th century. The discovery of the Assam tea variant of the *Camellia sinensis* plant was serendipitous. Soon, the British established vast plantations, with Assam and Darjeeling becoming synonymous with fine tea.

Spreading the Seed: Africa and Beyond

India was but a chapter in Britain's tea tale. Colonies in Kenya, Malawi, and South Africa soon found themselves amidst tea plantations. Africa, with its conducive climate, swiftly rose to be one of the largest producers globally.

Cultural Cups: Tea's Impact on Societies

Every nation that tea touched, it transformed. In Russia, it led to the birth of the Samovar tea culture. In the Middle East, it became an emblem of hospitality. And in the Americas, it symbolized rebellion – the Boston Tea Party stands testament.

Tea, in essence, was never just about the brew. It was a reflection of geopolitics, cultural amalgamations, and evolving global dynamics.

A Spiritual Steep: The Ethereal Essence of Tea

Zen and the Tea Ceremony

In the bamboo-filled alcoves of Japan, the way of tea, or *Chanoyu*, emerged not just as a ceremony but as an embodiment of Zen Buddhism. It wasn't about the tea itself, but the act of preparation and the quest for simplicity and purity. In this singular act of preparing Matcha, the powdered green tea, the monks sought to unify mind, body, and spirit. To be in the moment, to appreciate the fleeting nature of life, and to find enlightenment in the mundane act of boiling water and whisking tea. The room, the utensils, the very movements of the tea master - each was a meditation, a step closer to spiritual oneness.

The Tao of Tea in China

Long before Japan, it was China where tea was considered a means to connect with the divine. Ancient Daoist texts saw it as a potion of immortality. It was no wonder that hermits and monks in the misty mountains of China treasured it. They believed that tea, when consumed in its pure form, had the power to purify the soul and provide clarity of thought, essential for meditation and spiritual introspection.

From Leaf to Life: Health Benefits Through the Ages

Green Tea: The Eastern Elixir

In China and Japan, green tea's medicinal qualities were celebrated. Traditional Chinese Medicine advocated its use for everything from treating headaches to dispelling toxins. It was seen as a balancer of the body's five elements. Green tea's antioxidants, notably EGCG, were believed to have the power to rejuvenate the skin, enhance longevity, and even aid in weight loss.

Black Tea: Vitality in a Cup

Moving westward, as green tea oxidized into black tea, so did its perceived health benefits. Rich in theaflavins and thearubigins, black tea was revered in ancient Tibetan monasteries for its supposed benefits to heart health and digestion. In the courts of England, it was often seen as a mild stimulant and a digestive aid after rich meals.

White Tea: Nature's Gentle Healer

The least processed of all teas, white tea, primarily from China's Fujian province, was reserved for the upper classes. The very finest white teas were considered so precious that they were suitable gifts for the emperor. Its delicate nature was believed to be beneficial for the skin and overall vitality. Rich in catechins, it was considered a tonic for youth and beauty.

The Global Goblet: Variations and Vestiges

Chai: India's Spiced Concoction

While the British introduced tea to India, India introduced the world to Chai. A fragrant brew of black tea, spices like cardamom, ginger, cloves, and milk, it became a staple across the subcontinent. Beyond its delicious taste, chai, with its medley of spices, was considered beneficial for digestion and a shield against the common cold.

Oolong: The Balance Beam

Straddling between green and black tea, Oolong, with its semi-oxidized leaves, offers a unique flavor profile and health benefits. Traditionally used in Chinese weight loss regimens, it is believed to boost metabolism and reduce cholesterol.

Sencha: The Steamed Delight of Japan

In the Land of the Rising Sun, Sencha, a type of green tea, stands as the most popular brew. Unlike its Chinese counterparts which are pan-fried, Sencha leaves are steamed, yielding a more vegetal and grassy flavor. Revered not just for its refreshing taste, it has also been a cornerstone of the Japanese tea ceremony, symbolizing peace, harmony, and happiness. Rich in antioxidants, it's been linked to potential benefits like enhancing brain function and protection against heart diseases.

Earl Grey: The Scented Gem of the West

Distinguished by its unique addition of oil from the rind of the bergamot orange, Earl Grey has become synonymous with British tea culture. Its fragrant citrusy aroma contrasts beautifully with the robustness of the black tea it is typically paired with. The name carries an aristocratic air, credited to Charles Grey, the 2nd Earl Grey and a former British Prime Minister. Historically, apart from its distinctive flavor, it's believed that the bergamot oil had qualities that aided digestion.

A Note of Caution: The Fine Line

While tea is a treasure trove of health benefits, moderation is key. Excessive consumption can lead to insomnia due to caffeine or even iron deficiency, particularly in the case of green tea. Over-steeping black tea can sometimes cause an upset stomach or jitteriness. But when consumed in balanced quantities, the benefits vastly outweigh the cons.

Concluding Leaves: The Universal Uplifter

Tea is an enigma. Simple leaves and water, yet deeply complex in aroma, taste, and significance. It has traveled through time, across empires, and into the very heart of diverse cultures. Each cup tells a tale, not just of regions or recipes, but of rituals, remedies, and reverences. It's more than a drink. It's a shared global heritage, a unifier, a testament to humanity's quest for health, happiness, and spiritual harmony.

Our Gift to You: Free eBooks Every Week

Dear reader,

As you journey through the annals of history with Hourglass History, we're both humbled and delighted to be your chosen guide. It's a path that we tread together, discovering stories and legacies that have shaped our world.

In the spirit of furthering this voyage of discovery, we've crafted a special offer for our dedicated readers: **Freebie Fridays**. By signing up to our Freebie Friday email list, you will receive just one email each week containing at least one free eBook from Hourglass History.

All we kindly ask in return? After you've delved into the pages and immersed yourself in the tales of yesteryears, please consider leaving us a review on Amazon. Your insights, thoughts, and feedback not only help us refine our offerings but also guide fellow readers on their own historical journeys.

Here's our promise to you:

1. **Quality Over Quantity:** Every book you receive will be one of our full-length books that we normally sell at our full prices.

2. **Privacy is Paramount:** We hold your trust in the highest regard. Rest assured, your details will remain confidential, always.

3. **No Unwanted Distractions:** Our communications will be limited to our one "Freebie Fridays" email each week. No spam. Ever.

4. **Freedom to Choose:** While we'd love to have you with us forever, should you decide to walk different paths, unsubscribing is simple and instant.

To be part of this unique journey, simply sign up at Hourglass History Freebie Fridays (https://hourglasshistory.com/freebie-fridays/), or scan the following QR code:

Your first free eBook is just a Friday away.

Beyond the Pages: Your Part in the Story

We've traveled vast landscapes, meandered through history, and delved deep into the botanical wonders of teas. From the bustling markets of the Middle East to the serene monasteries of Asia, we've shared tales, discoveries, and the undying legacy of herbal teas. Now, as we come to the conclusion of this journey, we want to invite you to play an integral part in our ongoing story.

The Power of Your Voice

Your perspective, experience, and feedback are invaluable. Your voice has the potential to inspire, guide, and connect with countless other herbal tea enthusiasts, history buffs, and avid readers around the world.

Sharing Your Experience

If this book has added value to your life, informed you about the wonders of herbal teas, or taken you on a memorable journey through time and cultures, we kindly ask you to consider sharing your experience.

A review on Amazon not only helps us understand what resonated with you but also assists others in discovering this treasure trove of stories and information. Your words could guide someone else on this enchanting journey.

Why Reviews Matter

1. **Discoverability:** With millions of titles available on Amazon, reviews help our book rise above the noise and reach more readers.

2. **Feedback Loop:** Your insights guide us. They inform future editions, other writings, and how we approach topics. We're in this journey together, and your feedback is the compass.

3. **Building a Community:** Every review, comment, or feedback fosters a community of like-minded individuals. It's a place where we can share, learn, and grow together, united by our love for tea, history, and storytelling.

A Simple Gesture, A Lasting Impact

Leaving a review takes just a few minutes, but its impact can be profound. You'll be helping us continue our work, reach more readers, and further the appreciation for the magical world of herbal teas.

How to Leave a Review on Amazon:

1. Visit the book's Amazon page.

2. Scroll down to the "Customer Reviews" section.

3. Click on "Write a customer review."

4. Rate the book and share your thoughts, experiences, and feedback.

From the depths of our hearts, thank you for being a part of this journey. We look forward to hearing from you, growing with you, and sipping many more cups of herbal tea with you.